Basic Surgical Techniques

The Author

R. M. KIRK, M.S., F.R.C.S.

Consultant Surgeon, Royal Free Hospital Group, London, N.W.3;
Consultant Surgeon, Willesden General Hospital, London, N.W. 10.

Basic Surgical Techniques

R. M. KIRK

CHURCHILL LIVINGSTONE
Edinburgh and London 1973

CHURCHILL LIVINGSTONE
Medical Division of Longman Group Limited

Represented in the United States of America by
Longman Inc., New York, and by associated
companies, branches and representatives throughout
the world

ISBN 0 443 01065 X

Set and composed by Print Origination, Liverpool
and printed offset by T. & A. Constable,
Hopetoun Street, Edinburgh

PREFACE

I have described the manual skills that are used during the performance of surgical operations but avoiding, as far as possible, reference to specific operations which are described in many excellent books.

It might be claimed that this form of instruction is best transmitted by a master surgeon to his apprentice in the operating theatre. I agree with this view. The man burning with a desire to become a surgeon will, in most countries, be superbly trained. He does not require textbooks of this type, though I suspect he will read it more avidly than most. However, there are many others who occasionally carry out surgical procedures, including physicians, dentists, veterinarians, and experimentalists who have not been given the long apprenticeship in operative technique, and this book is aimed at them. The pressure of circumstances may make surgeons of most doctors once they leave highly developed urban communities.

Experienced surgeons enjoy reading of surgical technique in the hope of learning, and of spotting omissions. I hope that the techniques I have described will be of interest to other surgeons. None of them are of my own invention. I owe them to my teachers whether these be revered masters, or young assistants.

It may appear incongruous that having written a book on operative skill I can declare that I do not excessively revere surgical technique, nor do I claim to be above average in my personal operative skill. The qualities that I do admire, and to which I aspire, are good judgment, and safe surgery. A fast knot does not impress me, but a safely tied one leaves me content. A surgeon can slickly insert a run of stitches that impresses his audience; he may know, and he is sometimes the only one to know, that they are imperfect. My aim in writing this book is not to inspire surgical virtuosi, but to promote careful, safe techniques and regard for the living tissues.

It is a pleasure to thank Mrs Joyce Lindsell for her outstanding skill and accuracy in preparing the typescript. Mr Frank Price has carried out some of the illustrations.

1973   R.M.KIRK

CONTENTS

Preface

To my parents

Chapter 1

HANDLING YOURSELF

Mental attitude

Most operators work best in a relaxed atmosphere of quiet calm resulting from confidence that they are competent to cope with the problems of the operation. Usually there is no urgency and each step can be undertaken deliberately.

Do not allow yourself to be thrown off balance by an unexpected disaster, anxiety generated by another member of the team, or the presence of a senior colleague. At such times pause momentarily to re-assess the whole situation, decide what to do and get on with it. The agony of indecisiveness that crumbles your self-confidence is best dispelled either by stopping the procedure completely, or continuing to perform some routine task, while thinking out the problem. Discussing and displaying the problem to other members of the team is particularly valuable—it does not matter if they cannot understand the technicalities. As you declare the problem, and the arguments in favour of the possible choices of action, you will help yourself to reach a decision.

It is fortunate that sheer panic is most unusual; errors are most frequently made because new events or findings are not incorporated into the operator's broad view of the procedure. Do not, when circumstances suddenly change, avoid taking a decision by doggedly and blindly pursuing the course of action that had been decided upon before the circumstances changed.

A few operators flourish only in an atmosphere of tension and drama. These colourful characters have become associated with the public view of surgeons in action. It is only their present day rarity that makes them noteworthy. Those of us who find such tension anathematous take great care to avoid them as colleagues.

1

Physical attitude

Many manoeuvres are best performed in a particular way, such as stitching with a straight needle pointed away from the body, cutting with a scalpel from left to right, and cutting with scissors from right to left. When performing in this fashion an operator feels and looks natural. Whenever possible, plan to perform manoeuvres in the easiest and most practised manner. Some surgeons who never appear clumsy, are skilful at arranging to operate always from an advantageous position.

You may avoid a difficult manoeuvre by re-aligning yourself in relation to the task. The ability to do this explains the unconscious adoption of a standing posture by many surgeons. Sometimes only a rotation of the shoulders suffices. At other times it may be necessary to walk to the opposite side of the table.

A physical change of posture is not always necessary. A mental realignment of the body or shoulders may demonstrate the best approach to the problem.

Inevitably there are occasions when, in spite of careful assessment of the difficulties, an unfamiliar manoeuvre is demanded and must be accepted. If it is necessary to tie a knot in an unfamiliar plane, take extra care to tie it and tighten it correctly. When placing stitches at unusual angles, try several methods of holding the needle, and select the one which produces the greatest control of the stitching.

It is difficult but sometimes necessary to use the scalpel to cut from right to left, or scissors to cut from left to right. Since the two important cutting instruments are normally used in opposite directions, consider exchanging one for the other to allow a controlled cut to be made.

Hands

If you have watched even a few surgeons at work, you will realize that there is no such thing as the ideal surgeon's hand. Some surgeons have long slim hands and fingers, others have broad hands, with short, thick, flat-ended fingers. The comparative lengths of fingers also differ. All of us have individual subconscious preferences for using our fingers when performing particular tasks. The ability to oppose fingers varies. The terminal phalanx and the shape of its covering pulp, skin, and nail alters the use of the fingers. Some fingers most easily press with their tips; fingers in which the nail bed extends to the tips most comfortably press with the palmar surface of the pulps. Some fingers have hyperextensible terminal interphalangeal joints, making pulp pressure easy, others have not, so that end pressure is easier.

Manual dexterity is not an essential for good technique. Some surgeons look slow and clumsy in their hand movements, yet the directness of their approach to the tasks more than makes up for this. Left handed people are at no disadvantage except that technical descriptions, as in this book, apply to right handed people since they form the majority of the population. However, left handed people are well adapted to living in a world where they form the minority, and they are able to transpose instructions with facility.

STABILITY. Surgeons do not have extraordinary steady hands. Everyone has a hand tremor. If you extend your hands and arms the tips of your outstretched fingers can be seen to shake slightly with each heartbeat. If you hold a long-handled instrument at arm's length the tremor is magnified at the tip of the instrument. Anxiety produces a variable increase in the tremor. Do not feel diffident about your ability to perform delicate surgical operations because you appear to have shaky hands, but learn to steady them against a firm base.

The steadiness of the hands is related to the distance from the steady base. When you stand with your hands extended in front of you, the ends of your fingers are at a great distance from the base formed by your feet. If you hold your elbows tightly against your sides this effectively shortens your arms and steadies your hands. If you sit, or brace your hips against a fixed object, your hands will become even steadier. Alternatively you may rest your elbows against a table. For very fine work, it may be possible to rest your wrist, or little finger against the table (Fig. 1) whilst using the thumb and lateral fingers to carry out a finely controlled movement.

If no other base can be used, the other hand may exert a steadying influence. The blades of scissors held in one hand may be rested against the outstretched fingers of the other hand (Fig. 2). It may be difficult to thread a needle, holding the thread in one hand and the needle in the other; this is facilitated by pressing together the wrists of both hands (Fig. 3). Sometimes an instrument may be rested against a firm structure, and the hand rests against this, like an artist using a mahl-stick.

When a finely controlled movement must be made, do not hesitate to practise it in the air. This is much used by artists and also by golfers.

3

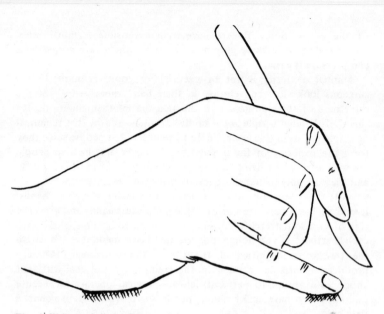

Fig. 1 Wrist and little finger used as a steadying bridge while holding the scalpel during precision cutting.

Assisting at operations

A single operator cannot always carry out several tasks simultaneously and many procedures require the assistance of one or more persons. Some operators, whether from choice or necessity,

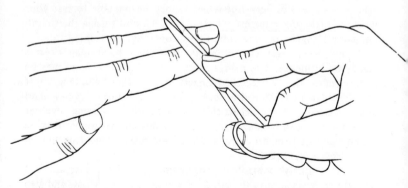

Fig. 2 Steadying an instrument against the fingers of the other hand.

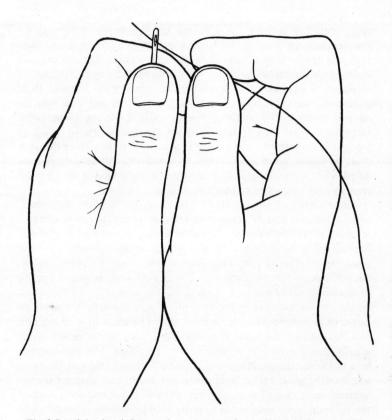

Fig. 3 Steadying hands by pressing wrists together whilst threading a needle.

become very skilled at performing complicated operations with little or no assistance.

Assisting at operations serves a second very important function, as a training ground for future surgeons. Do not look upon assisting someone else as a necessary boring prelude to carrying out the procedure yourself. The privilege of assisting a skilled operator allows you to acquire judgment and technique both consciously and unconsciously, so that when you come to perform the procedure yourself, you will automatically adopt safe and effective techniques.

If you are to assist in carrying out an unfamiliar operation, read up the anatomy beforehand, so that you can mentally perform the steps with the surgeon, anticipating his needs. However, restrain your enthusiasm from trying to take over the operation. Remember that the operator primarily requires from you the display, in good light, of the structures on which the operation is being performed.

Fall into step with the atmosphere required by the surgeon. Most operators like to maintain a relaxed atmosphere and you may be allowed to ask questions during routine parts of the operation. Some surgeons like to work quietly without distraction. There are times when it is important to recognize that an important step or decision must be taken, when any surgeon would resent chit-chat. If you are asked your opinion, give it honestly and be prepared to give the reasons which lead you to that conclusion.

Sometimes you see something you think the surgeon has missed, or you consider that he is about to make an error. Do not hesitate to mention it. If the surgeon continues as before, remember that the final decision must be his. Do not indulge in an argument over the propriety of the action. This does not preclude you from subsequently asking him to discuss his action with you, provided you do so at an opportune moment.

Do not be disloyal to the surgeon. If you think he has made an error, or is incompetent, learn from the experience of working with him but do not denigrate him. We learn from all those we assist, usually positive lessons of how best to do things, but also learning how not to do things. It is possible that with increasing maturity you will modify your earlier judgments and blush with shame over the ignorant arrogance of some of them. Perhaps the commonest fault of the inexperienced assistant is to be dazzled by technical mastery and not sufficiently appreciate the importance of good judgment.

You may be fortunate enough to be delegated parts of the operation. In your enthusiasm do not select speed as the paramount quality with which to impress the surgeon; he will be more willing to give you increased responsibility if you display carefulness and calmness. However, if you are likely to be allowed to take an active part, prepare yourself by becoming competent at simple mechanical skills such as knot-tying and the handling of instruments. It is intensely annoying to be inveigled into giving a pressing assistant a task, only to find that he has not bothered to prepare for it.

As you become more competent and as you are given more personal responsibility you will learn even more from assisting than formerly, since you will be aware of more of the problems. You may then be awarded the privileged relationship with the surgeon of being treated on equal terms while the finer points are discussed and demonstrated. You will later, when you are the operator, realize how much it is appreciated to discuss the problem with an assistant who is aware of it, and the dilemma which it presents. The solution which is mutually arrived at, will be a source of satisfaction and a lesson for the future if it proves correct, and the arguments which led to it will be a solace if it proves incorrect.

Chapter 2

HANDLING INSTRUMENTS

Modern surgical instruments have reached near perfection from constant improvements by surgeons and manufacturers. Treat them with great care.

For most purposes a limited range of standard instruments is adequate. Learn to use these well before demanding specialized instruments.

Scalpel

Use this for making deliberate cuts in tissues, dividing them with the minimum of trauma. The scalpel is most commonly used for incising skin, for dissecting connective tissues covering the area which is to be displayed, and for deliberately dividing a structure.

In order to cut with the minimum tissue damage, draw the whole length of the sharp blade, not merely the point, over the tissues. If the edge is pressed upon the tissues, cutting is inefficient and uncontrolled. The combination of drawing the knife and controlled pressure, determines the depth of cut.

The method of holding the knife varies according to the use which is made of it. For cutting skin and similar tissues, grasp the handle in a similar manner to that for holding a table knife (Fig. 4). Keep the knife horizontal, suspended beneath the pronated hand, held between thumb and middle finger. The index finger pulp lies upon the back of the knife at the base of the blade. The ring and little fingers reinforce the control of the middle finger. The end of the handle rests against the medial edge of the hand. For delicate division of fine structures, hold the knife like a pen (Fig. 1).

Do not use the scalpel for cutting unsuitable structures such as metal or bone. Cartilage may be cut with a heavy type of scalpel which is usually kept for the purpose. Do not use a blunt scalpel. If

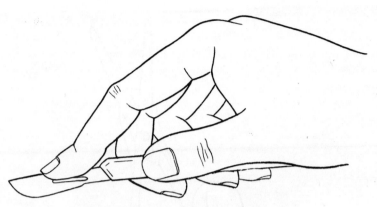

Fig. 4 Holding the scalpel for cutting skin.

part of the cutting edge is lost, cutting will be uneven, more pressure must be applied, and control is lost.

Do not cut until you have assessed the situation. It may be possible to repair most cuts, but a few are irretrievable. Occasionally it is worth practising in the air, like a golfer preparing to putt, before making a long, clean scalpel cut.

If an important structure lies in the line of the proposed cut protect it, whenever possible, by interposing an instrument between the tissues to be cut and the vital structure. The closed blades of dissecting forceps, a grooved dissector, or a probe, can sometimes be inserted in the line of the cut, beneath the tissue to be divided, protecting the important structure.

When a cut must be performed at some depth from the surface, a bistoury may be used. This is a long, thin-bladed knife, sharp tipped for end cutting, probe pointed for side cutting. The bistoury is occasionally combined with a grooved dissector for cutting through a bridge of tissue running vertically from the surface. Whenever possible, improve the display so that the dissection can be performed with an ordinary scalpel.

Scissors

The cutting action results from the moving edge-contact between the blades which are given a slight set towards each other. Except for special uses, sharp-pointed scissors are not used in surgery; the ends are usually chamfered for dissection and general purposes, and blunt-nosed for ligature cutting.

9

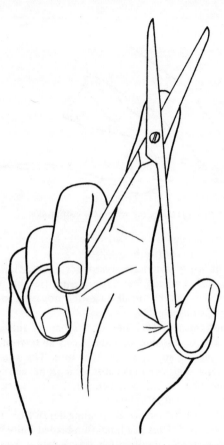

Fig. 5 Holding scissors.

Insert the thumb in one ring of the handle; this will be the moving blade. Insert the middle, ring or little finger into the other ring, and curl the other two fingers round the outside of the ring to steady it; this will be the fixed blade. Place the index finger pulp on the joint to steady it (Fig. 5).

The hand is usually most comfortable when held midway between pronation and supination, especially when cutting from right to left. When cutting down a hole the tips may be more easily visible with the hand held in supination. Exceptionally the scissors may be held pointing towards the body, alongside, and parallel to

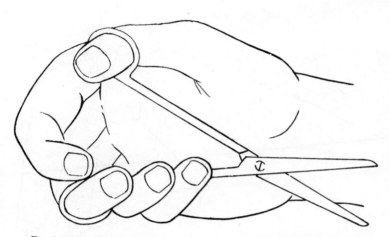

Fig. 6 Cutting from left to right whilst holding scissors in the right hand.

the fore-arm when cutting from left to right, unless you are ambidextrous (Fig. 6).

Always press upon the handles so that the blades are kept in contact with each other. If they spring apart the cutting action is replaced by tearing. For this reason never use scissors that are too fine for the work, or the blades will be forced apart.

For rather snobbish reasons scissors were formerly despised as dissecting instruments, the scalpel being favoured. In some circumstances scissors are greatly to be preferred.

Dissecting forceps (thumb forceps)

These forceps grip when compressed between thumb and fingers (Fig. 7). When released, the blades spring apart because the springy steel from which they are made is given a set during manufacture. Delicate forceps have a pointed post on the inner side of one blade which engages a hole in the opposite blade, to maintain the opposition of the tips.

These forceps are ideal for giving a changing and temporary grasp of tissues. They usually have no lock for maintaining the grip.

Two main types of dissecting forceps are available, toothed and non-toothed. The toothed variety usually has a single central spur on the tip of one blade, interdigitating with two spurs on the other blade. The tissue is held by the teeth punctures rather than by compression between the blades. For this reason, delicate tissues are

11

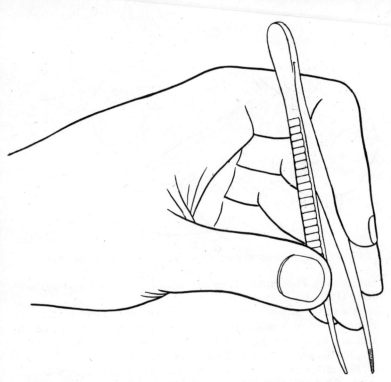

Fig. 7 Gripping dissecting forceps. Notice that the left hand is being used.

sometimes less injured if grasped with toothed forceps than if grasped with the non-toothed variety. Very tough slippery tissues can be firmly gripped with heavy toothed forceps. Toothed forceps may have, in addition, roughened areas near the teeth to improve the grip.

Non-toothed forceps depend for their holding power on serrations of the apposing surfaces of the tips, and upon the strength of the grip. When selecting dissecting forceps, favour those that require the least gripping force to control the tissues. Small ducts, blood vessels, skin, fascia, cartilage, and bone are gripped with toothed forceps of increasing heaviness through the list. Peritoneum, bowel, liver and other encapsulated solid organs are usually picked up with non-toothed forceps, to avoid puncturing them.

Never select forceps that are too fragile for the intended purpose. If you do, they will not grip efficiently, the tips may be strained out

12

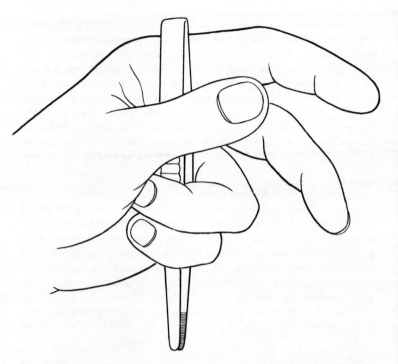

Fig. 8 Palming the dissecting forceps to free the thumb, index and middle fingers.

of alignment and the forceps are ruined. Never select forceps that are too heavy for the task, because they will damage the tissues. Do not apply dissecting forceps at one point for too long, or the tissues will become crushed and necrotic. Do not use dissecting forceps to apply continuous traction. Select tissue forceps, hooks, or retractors.

Learn to manipulate dissecting forceps with the left hand (Fig. 7). They form an excellent multipurpose instrument for displaying structures during dissection, whilst holding a scalpel or scissors in the right hand. They may be used with the blades closed as a gentle retractor, or to tense a loose structure that is to be cut. They grasp, display and test the tissues. Learn also to 'palm' them, holding them with the ring and little fingers, thus freeing the thumb and other fingers for grasping needles and tying knots (Fig. 8).

The closed blades of round-nosed, non-toothed forceps make an

13

excellent dissector. Insert them in the desired plane and their springiness gently opens up the plane. Sometimes the forceps may be gently pushed along, acting as a wedge that splits fragile overlying tissues. Sometimes the tip of the deep blade of a slightly opened pair of scissors can be trapped in the gap between the forceps blades away from their apposed tips, and the two instruments are pushed along, splitting open the track. Alternatively use a scalpel to divide the overlying tissue, aiming to cut between the forceps blades. In tissues too fine to be felt with the fingers, dissecting forceps give the operator his sense of feel to test the structures he meets.

Artery forceps (haemostatic forceps)

These forceps work with a scissors action and incorporate a ratchet lock and spring steel handles. The joint may be a simple one, or may be a beautifully constructed box joint, in which one blade passes through a channel formed in the other blade. The handles end in rings or bows through which fingers are inserted, like scissors. The rings allow pressure to be exerted in all directions from within the rings, to open and close the blades.

Many designs of straight or curved artery forceps are available, from delicate 'mosquito' forceps to heavy Kocher's tooth-ended

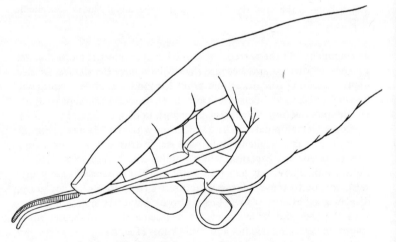

Fig. 9 Applying artery forceps.

forceps. The design makes them versatile. They make excellent dissectors for opening up tissue planes and tracks. They double up as tissue forceps, needle holders, knot-holding forceps, foreign body extractors, sinus forceps, and stitch-removing forceps.

APPLYING ARTERY FORCEPS. Insert the thumb into one ring, the little finger into the other ring which is also steadied by the middle and ring fingers. Place the index finger pulp on the forceps joint (Fig. 9). Be prepared to hold the hand in pronation or supination.

Grasp small vessels with the tips of the forceps. For larger vessels, try to pick up the vessel just proximal to the forceps points; this leaves a small projection of the tips of the forceps which facilitates the subsequent tying of a ligature. For a small vessel, one click of the ratchet suffices. For a major vessel, tighten the grip, listening for the clicks of the ratchet lock. Do not overtighten or the ratchet will over-run, allowing the forceps to spring off when they are released. Lay the forceps down with the handles towards the periphery of the wound.

Artery forceps are designed so that the tips oppose first. Therefore, pick up small pieces of tissue with the tips. Larger pieces of tissue should be grasped nearer the joint, or the forceps will be strained.

REMOVING ARTERY FORCEPS. Learn to control the forceps with either hand. For the right hand, hold the forceps in the same manner as described when applying them. For the left hand, firmly grasp the ring which presents to your left side, or the farthest from you, between the thumb on top or to your right, opposed by the index and middle fingers (Fig. 10). This becomes the fixed blade. Control the other (moving) blade with the pulps of the ring and little fingers hooked round the portion of the ring nearest the midline of the forceps.

The ratchet cannot be released until the spring handles have been compressed further. As you do this, control the forceps to ensure that they do not spring open. Separate the handles in a plane at right angles to the plane of action of the joint. If the handles were compressed sufficiently, there will be no click as the ratchet opens. Separate the handles while maintaining the strain on them, so preventing other segments of the ratchet from catching. If a ligature is being tied, release the grip just as the ligature begins to bite.

When assisting an operator to ligature clipped vessels, allow him to extend his arms, hands separated, ligature thread stretched

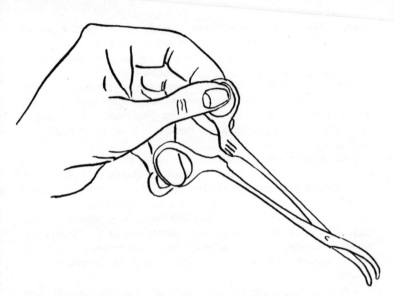

Fig. 10 Removing artery forceps with the left hand.

between his hands, to your side of the table. Reach over the stretched thread to pick up the handles of the artery forceps. Alternatively, gently lift the handles, allowing the operator to pass the end of the thread behind the forceps. As ligatures are tied round small vessels held in curved artery forceps, gently lower the handles so the convexity of the blades faces downwards, and the points face upwards. This allows the operator to run the thread beneath the point. As the ligature is tied, gently push the forceps in the direction of the points, to trap the thread.

When tying an important vessel with a double ligature, gently release the forceps as the first ligature is tightened, then reclamp it. As the second ligature is tightened, remove the forceps.

If the ligature encircles the tips of the forceps and not the vessel, the forceps blades cannot be opened. Do not forcibly overcome the resistance, or pull the forceps out of the ring of encircling ligature.

Report to the operator, and allow him to resite the ligature.

Never use short-handled artery forceps in the depths of large wounds, for fear of leaving them. Always use forceps with handles long enough to protrude through the wound. Check the numbers carefully before and after each procedure.

16

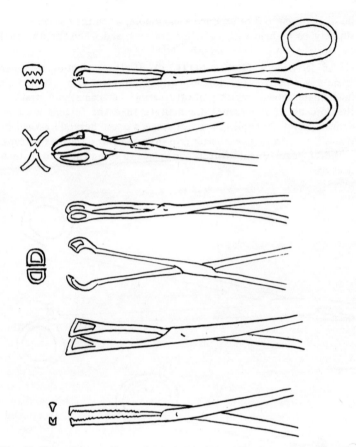

Fig. 11 Tissue forceps. From above downwards: Allis, Lane, ring, Babcock, Duval and Kocher.

Tissue forceps

These forceps rely for their grip on the shape and area of blade in contact with the tissue (Fig. 11), the roughness of the opposing surfaces, interlocking teeth, sharp hooked blades, or a combination of these. Some have ring-like blades, through which the tissues bulge and are thus held. These forceps have rachet handles so that they maintain their grip.

Tissue forceps are preferable whenever traction sutures or a sharp

17

hook might cut out or produce a leaky hole, when the tissues are too slippery to be held with smooth retractors, and when the direction of traction must be frequently varied.

CARE IN USING TISSUE FORCEPS. If strong traction of tough tissues is required, use forceps with a powerful grip, rather than inadequate forceps which pull off, tearing the tissues, and straining the forceps. If the tissues are delicate then the forceps must be delicate, carefully applied, and not dragged upon. Several lightweight tissue forceps may give a better grip than one pair of heavier forceps.

Never leave tissue forceps in place a moment longer than necessary.

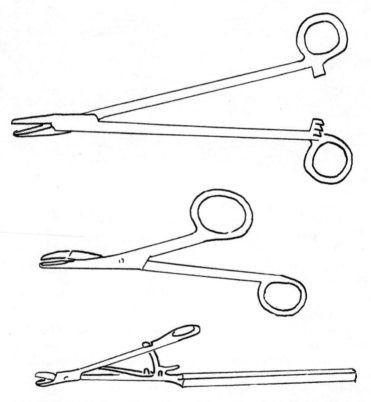

Fig. 12 Needle holders. From above downwards: Mayo, Gillies combined needleholder and suture scissors, and ophthalmic needle holder.

Needle holders

Straight needles are usually, though not inevitably, held in the fingers. Large curved needles may similarly be used in the hand. Small needles are nearly always curved and are best held in needle holders.

Needle holders (Fig. 12) grip the needle between specially designed jaws, and they may incorporate a ratchet lock so that they maintain their grip by the tension in the spring handles. Long-handled needle holders facilitate inserting sutures within deep cavities.

Needle holders are designed to be rotated in their long axis, since a pronation/supination action is used to drive a curved needle through the tissues. Some needle holders incorporate gripping surfaces designed to take needles at unusual angles, when suturing in restricted spaces.

Mayo's type needle holder is the simplest model and is used in many modifications. The action is similar to that of artery forceps but the handles are longer and the blades shorter in proportion.

Select the correct needle holder for the work. For delicate close stitching choose a fine short-handled needle holder. When stitching in the depths of a wound select a long-handled needle holder, so that the hand is outside the wound, not blocking the entrance. This allows light to reach the depths, and a view to be obtained as the stitches are inserted.

Retractors

These usefully hold aside tissues to expose deeper structures (Fig. 13). Some retractors are hand-held by an assistant and if properly used they cause minimal damage since the assistant relaxes tension on the tissues except when the operator requires display of the deep structure.

Self-retaining retractions may produce excellent exposure. They must be carefully placed and opened carefully to avoid damage to the tissue.

Clamps

A wide variety of instruments are used for grasping, joining, or compressing structures. The opposing faces and heaviness of the jaws differ, depending upon the purpose for which they will be used (Fig. 14). The mechanisms for fixing the clamps vary from spring handles with ratchet catches, to screw threads.

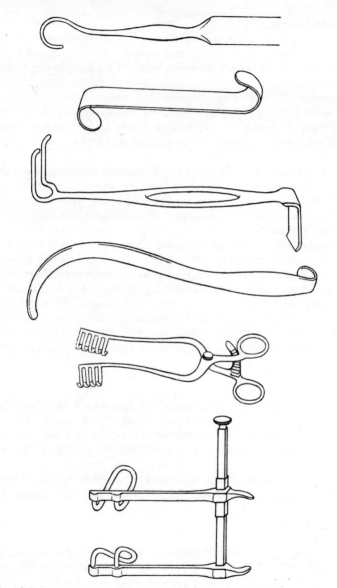

Fig. 13 Retractors. From above downwards: hook, malleable copper, Czerny, Deaver, self-retaining and Gosset self-retaining.

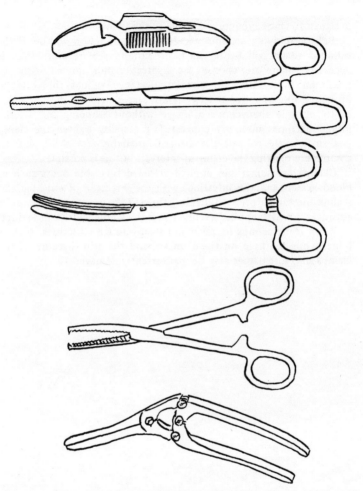

Fig. 14 Above, three non-crushing clamps: 'bulldog', Pott's arterial, and intestinal. Below, two crushing clamps: Kocher's arterial, and Payr's lever action intestinal.

Some clamps, as for instance artery forceps, are intended to crush and retain a grip of the grasped structure. The jaws are therefore strong and ridged to improve the grip. On the other hand clamps placed across deformable ducts to temporarily occlude them, are deliberately made with lightweight jaws. The opposing faces are also

21

designed to cause minimum damage to the tissues.

Before applying a clamp decide what its function will be. If the clamped tissue will be retained, do not damage it more than is necessary, therefore choose the lightest clamp applied with the minimum force. Only in one circumstance should this rule be broken. Soft tissue isolated by clamps placed across it in such a way as to occlude the venous drainage without stopping the arterial inflow becomes intensely congested; preferably tighten the clamp just sufficiently to halt the arterial circulation for short periods, completely relaxing the clamp at intervals, if this is possible.

Clamps are sometimes applied across deformable ducts such as blood vessels and the intestine, with the intention of crushing and sealing the lumen prior to dividing them. Take care to use clamps of adequate strength applied evenly across the whole width of the duct.

When using clamps to grasp and steady tough structures, such as bone, while working on them, make sure the grip is secure. If the clamps slip, soft tissues may be inadvertently damaged.

Chapter 3

HANDLING THREADS

Threads of various materials are extensively used during surgical operations for ligating (binding), and suturing (sewing). Almost in no other human activity does the manually dexterous person demonstrate his adroitness more clearly than when handling threads.

Most of the threads used in surgery, including catgut, are given a 'lay' or twist during manufacture, to hold the components together. If you hold one end of the thread and rotate the other end between finger and thumb (Fig. 15) to tighten the twist, the thread will form itself into a loop provided there is sufficient slack. Reverse the twist and the thread will straighten. If you twist it the other way, the thread may form a loop in the opposite direction or it may simply untwist. Loops made in this way do not require to be held but loops made by deforming the thread without regard to the lay will spring undone when they are released. When forming loops in heavier twisted threads, it becomes essential to take notice of the lay, as will be evident if a seaman is watched while he coils a rope.

Untwisted threads, such as monofilament nylon and wire, or braided threads, must be given a twist when looping them, otherwise the loop springs apart, or forms a kink which weakens the thread and may produce a snag. Twists are prone to build up during continuous suturing. When using springy material such as wire, delegate an assistant to control it to prevent kinking, and periodically run a flexible thread between finger and thumb from fixed end to free end to unwind the twists.

Loops of thread have an almost fiendish propensity to catch around the handles of surgical instruments and any other obstructions. To avoid this, remove all unnecessary instruments from the field, cover the handles of essential instruments, throw loops of thread clear of likely snags and detail an assistant to control the loops of thread.

23

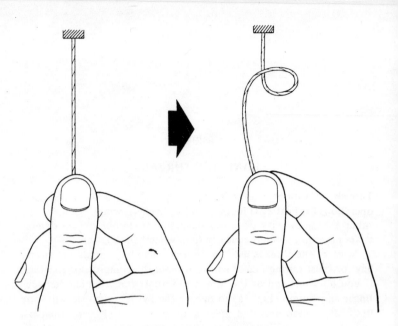

Fig. 15 Effect of twisting thread.

Select the correct size and texture of thread and if you are unsure seek advice. All threads inserted into living tissue evoke a reaction, so the smaller the amount, and the thinner, the better. However, the thread must be strong enough to hold. Remember that the force you exert in handling it must vary according to the tensile strength of the particular thread. Too strong a pull will either break the thread, or so weaken it that it will subsequently break. Remember that friction weakens the thread, so avoid dragging it over sharp edges.

Threads are fastened by knotting. Knots kink the thread and weaken it, and also form a source of weakness from slipping of the threads if they are not tightened sufficiently to bind against each other.

Knots

A knot is an intertwining of threads for the purpose of fastening them. The ends of ligatures and sutures are knotted together. Secure fastening results from friction between threads and this is affected by the area of contact, the thread surface, and the tightness of the knot.

24

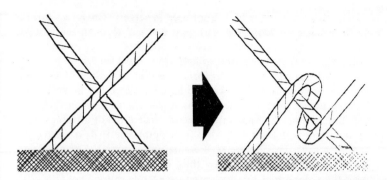

Fig. 16 Forming a half hitch.

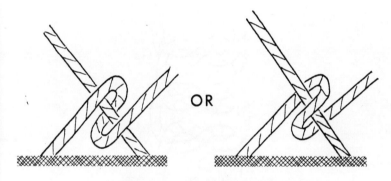

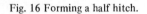

Fig. 17 Two types of half hitch: starting left over right or right over left.

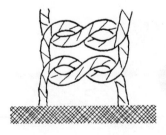

Fig. 18 Granny knot.

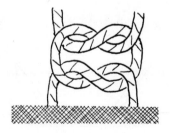

Fig. 19 Reef knot.

The half hitch is the basic knot used in surgery. Cross two threads to form a closed loop (Fig. 16); pass one end through the loop. A half hitch may be formed by crossing one thread over or under the other, thus making two forms of half hitch possible (Fig. 17).

After tying one half hitch, form a second half hitch of the same type to produce a granny knot (Fig. 18), which has much greater holding power than a single half hitch. Alternatively, after tying one half hitch, form the ends into a second half hitch of different type, producing a reef knot (Fig. 19) (reef points are tied to reduce the area of a sail). This has better holding power than the granny knot. After tying a reef knot, form a third half hitch, making a reef knot with the second half hitch, to produce a triple throw knot (Fig. 20). This is the most reliable knot of all. It is the standard knot used in surgery.

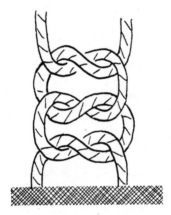

Fig. 20 Triple throw knot.

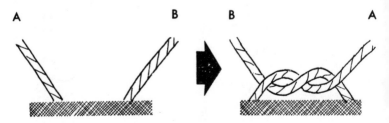

Fig. 21 When forming a half hitch, the ends must be crossed.

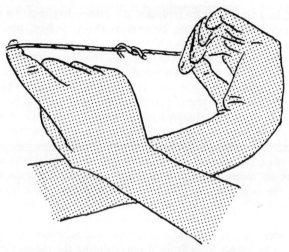

Fig. 22 Hands crossed in the horizontal plane.

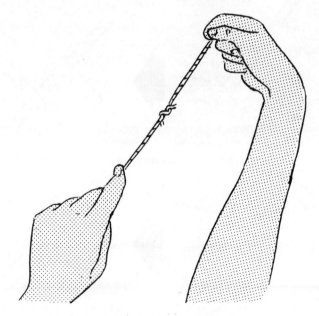

Fig. 23 Hands tying knot in the sagittal plane.

27

If two ends are to be tied in a half hitch, they must be crossed and tightened on the opposite sides of the knot from which they started (Fig. 21). The hands which control the ends must either cross each other, or exchange ends. If the hands are crossed in the horizontal plane after the manner of crossing hands at the pianoforte (Fig. 22), they obscure the knot as they cross. If the hands pass each other in the sagittal plane, towards and away from the body (Fig. 23), the knot is not obscured at any time. You may be able to tie knots in the sagittal plane by adjusting your posture, either physically or mentally.

A half hitch may be tied in one of two ways. In the first way, the threads are crossed to form a closed loop and one end is then passed under the crossing (Fig. 24). Both hands take an active part in the formation of the loop and the passing of the thread in a two handed knot. In a one handed knot, only one hand actively forms the loop and passes the end. The other end of thread is held passively either in the other hand or in an instrument during the formation of the

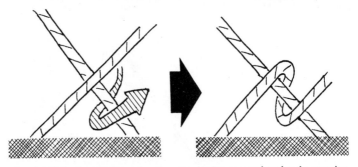

Fig. 24 Tying knot by crossing threads, passing one end under the crossing.

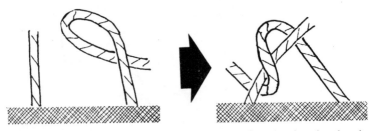

Fig. 25 Tying knot by forming loop in one thread and passing the other thread through the loop.

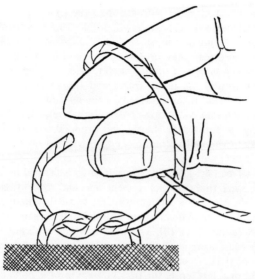

Fig. 26 Tying a half hitch by grasping one thread through a loop formed in the other thread.

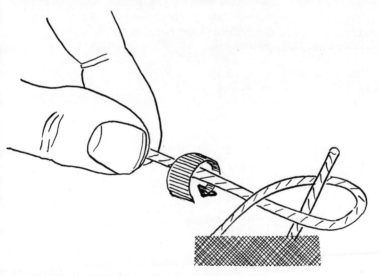

Fig. 27 Tying a half hitch by throwing a loop formed in one thread over the end of the other thread.

knot, although it must be moved during the tightening of the knot.

In the second way of tying a half hitch, a loop is formed in one thread and the end of the other thread is passed through the loop (Fig. 25). One thread may be carried in a complete turn around the jaws of forceps such as a needle holder, artery forceps or dissecting forceps, or around the index finger and thumb of one hand. The other end of thread is then grasped by the instrument or fingers, and drawn through the loop (Fig. 26). Alternatively, the loop in one thread may be formed in the air and dropped over the end of the other thread. The end is then picked up with an instrument or the fingers (Fig. 27).

FAULTS IN TYING KNOTS. If a half hitch is formed by one thread around another thread which is held taut and straight, the hitch is able to slide along the straight thread. If further half hitches are thrown in the same manner, while still holding the same thread taut, a slip knot results (Fig. 28). The way in which the knot is laid and tightened is just as important in producing a secure fastening as the formation of the correct hitches.

If the knot is left loose, the friction between the parts of thread is reduced and the knot fails to secure the ends. As the knot is tightened, the direction of pull on the threads must be along a straight line which passes through the centre of the knot. Any other direction of pull displaces the knot and puts traction on the tissues to which the knot is fastened.

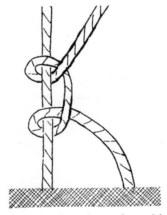

Fig. 28 Faulty knot. Half hitches formed around a straight taut thread produce a slip knot.

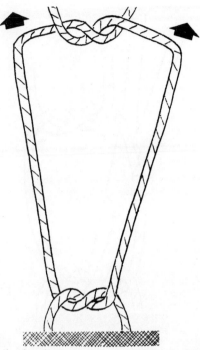

Fig. 29 Tying knots under tension. After tightening the first half hitch the threads are kept taut while the second half hitch is formed.

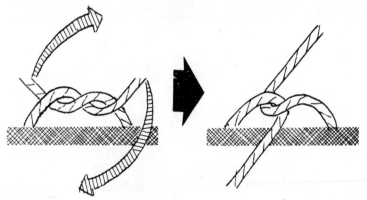

Fig. 30 Tying knots under tension. After tightening the first half hitch, it is jammed by rotating the threads, while the second half hitch is formed.

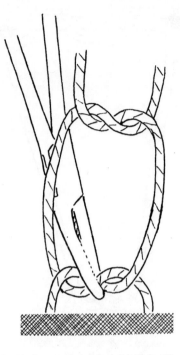

Fig. 31 Tying knots under tension. After tightening the first half hitch, it is grasped by forceps while the second half hitch is formed.

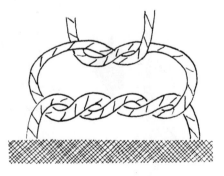

Fig. 32 Tying knots under tension. A surgeon's knot has an extra turn in the first half hitch.

DIFFICULTIES IN TYING KNOTS. If knots have to be tied in threads which draw together two structures under tension, avoid letting the first half hitch slip while forming the second. After tightening the first half hitch, keep a little tension on the threads while forming and tightening the second half hitch (Fig. 29). Alternatively, having tightened the first half hitch by pulling the threads in the correct line, sharply rotate them to jam the first half hitch (Fig. 30), while the second hitch is formed. As the second half hitch is tightened, the jammed threads are automatically released.

The assistant's finger may be pressed on the tightened first half hitch; the second hitch is formed and tightened onto it beneath the trapping finger, which is gently lifted. Alternatively an assistant may be asked to grasp the first half hitch with forceps after it has been tightened, to prevent it from loosening while the second half hitch is formed (Fig. 31). The assistant must release the grasp of the forceps on the first half hitch just as the second hitch is tightened upon it. A surgeon's knot may be tied to prevent the first half hitch from slipping. The end is carried a second time under the loop of the first half hitch (Fig. 32). When this is tightened, the friction of the extra turn is sufficient to prevent the hitch from slipping. A second half hitch is insufficient to secure the knot so a third half hitch must be tied, forming a reef knot with the second.

TYING KNOTS IN CAVITIES. In some situations it is easier to form the half hitch in a large loop outside the mouth of the cavity and tighten this, than to form a half hitch in the depths of the cavity (Fig. 33). Ensure that you have an adequate length of thread.

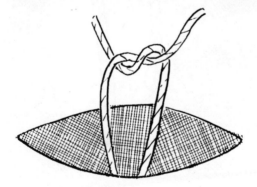

Fig. 33 Tying a knot in a cavity. The half hitch is formed outside instead of being tied in the depths.

When tightening the knot within the cavity, it is not always possible to pull the threads in opposite directions in the horizontal plane, yet they must be tightened by pulling in opposite directions. Try pushing one thread deeper into the cavity, while pulling the other thread towards the surface (Fig. 34).

STIFF OR SPRINGY MATERIAL. Stiff material is difficult to tie into a knot and thereafter to tighten. Stainless steel wire thread may kink if it is not guided as it is tightened. Get your assistant to place a smooth metal instrument under each half hitch to guide the run of the thread, withdrawing the instrument as the hitch tightens.

Springy ligature material, such as monofilament nylon, may loosen after the knot has been tightened, particularly if there is subsequently any movement in the tissues. To prevent this, tighten

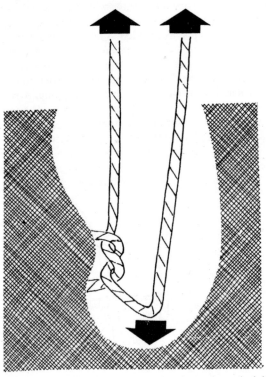

Fig. 34 Tightening a knot in a cavity. One thread may be pushed deeper into the cavity, while traction is exerted upon the other thread.

several more half hitches formed as reef knots in relationship to each other, to secure the deeper ones from slipping.

GENERAL ADVICE. Tie knots with unfailing accuracy. Quick but failed attempts are in the end slower. Moreover, at times there is no second chance.

Learn one method of tying for each situation. Practise the movements until they can be reproduced faultlessly.

METHODS OF FORMING KNOTS. It is often convenient to have one long and one short end when tying a knot, since an end must be passed through a loop or under a crossing of threads. The best methods of knot tying ensure that the end is always controlled during the passage through the loop or under the crossing.

Many ingenious methods have been described for tying knots. Only a few can be mentioned here, but they are all useful in certain circumstances, so learn them all. You may see someone using variations which you find suit your personal hand movements better than standard methods. For general use, employ two hands as you would tie shoe laces since this is the quickest and surest method.

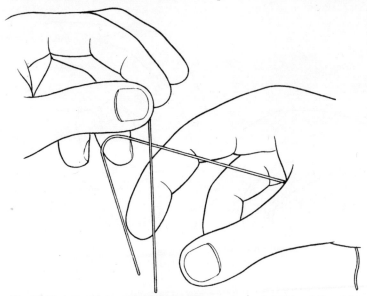

Fig. 35 The ring finger of the left hand draws a loop of right hand thread behind the short end held by the left hand. The crossing of the threads is about to be trapped by the pronated right hand between the index finger and thumb.

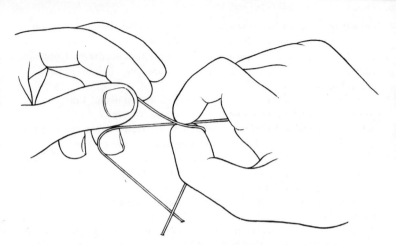

Fig. 36 The fully pronated right hand has trapped the crossing of the threads between the thumb and index finger. The left hand is about to release the short end of thread.

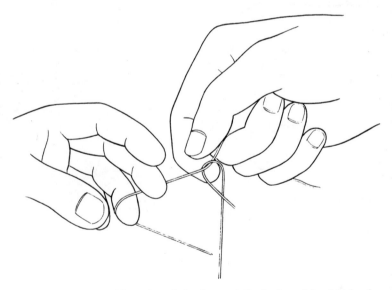

Fig. 37 The left hand has released the short end. Supination of the right hand has carried the short end under the crossing of the threads where it will again be grasped by the left hand.

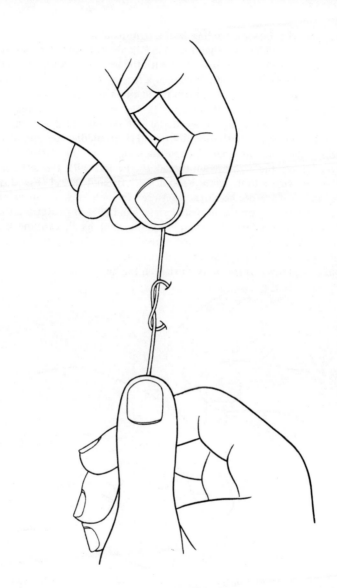

Fig. 38 The left hand takes one short end away from the body, the right hand takes the long end towards the body, to tighten the knot.

However, you may be holding in the right hand an instrument, such as a needle holder, so that this hand holds one thread passively, while a one-handed knot is formed with the left hand. An alternative would be to use the needle holder or a forceps to tie the knot. Even if you are not ambidextrous, learn to tie knots with either hand.

Two handed knot, Method 1. If the short end of thread is towards you, pick it up between the left thumb and index finger. Grip the longer end with the fully flexed right middle, ring and little fingers, allowing the spare thread to hang from the curled little finger. Hook the right hand thread to the left with the left ring finger, drawing a loop across behind the left hand thread (Fig. 35). Trap the crossing of the threads between the pulp of the right index finger and thumb of the pronated right hand (Fig. 36). Release the left hand thread, and fully supinate the right hand, carrying the short end under the crossing of threads (Fig. 37). Grasp the end again with the left hand and take it away from the body as the right hand moves towards the body to tighten the hitch (Fig. 38).

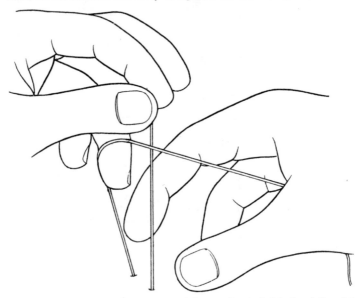

Fig. 39 The ring finger of the left hand draws a loop of right hand thread in front of the short end held by the left hand. The crossing of the threads is about to be trapped by the supinated right hand between the index finger and thumb.

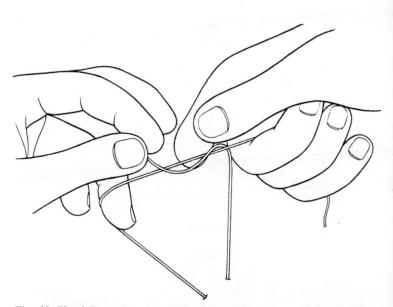

Fig. 40 The fully supinated right hand traps the crossing of the threads between index finger and thumb. The left hand is about to release the short end of thread.

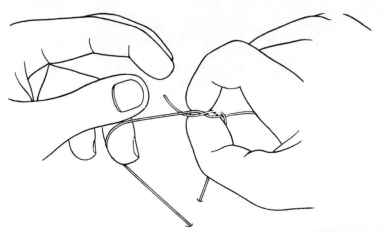

Fig. 41 The left hand has released the short end. The right hand is fully pronated, carrying the short end under the crossing of the threads where it will again be grasped by the left hand.

39

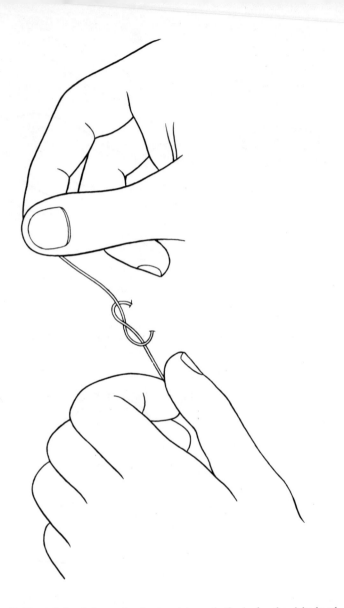

Fig. 42 The left hand draws the short end towards the body, the right hand draws the long thread away from the body to tighten the knot.

If the short end of the thread is away from you, pick it up with the left hand. Grip the longer thread with the fully flexed middle, ring and little fingers of the right hand, letting the spare thread hang from the curled little finger. Hook the right hand thread to the left with the left ring finger, across the front of the left hand thread (Fig. 39). Trap the crossing of the threads between the thumb and index finger of the fully supinated right hand (Fig. 40). Release the left hand thread, and fully pronate the right hand to carry the end under the crossing of the threads (Fig. 41). Grasp the end again with the left hand and bring it towards you as the right hand moves away to tighten the hitch (Fig. 42).

Two handed knot, Method 2. If the short end of thread is furthest from you, hold it vertically between the left thumb and index finger. Trap the longer end with the fully flexed middle, ring and little fingers of the right hand, allowing the spare thread to hang

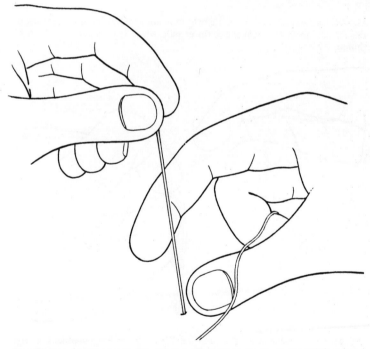

Fig. 43 Two handed knot. The short end is held vertically in the left hand and is about to be encircled by the right index finger.

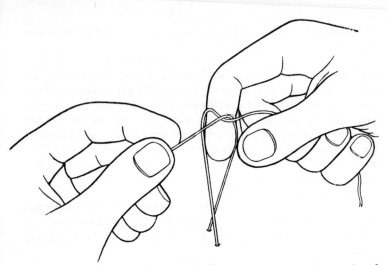

Fig. 44 Two handed knot. The right hand is supinated to bring the crossing of the threads on to the right index finger pulp where it is trapped by the right thumb.

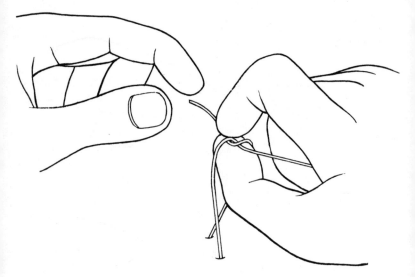

Fig. 45 Two handed knot. The right hand is pronated, carrying the short end under the crossing of the threads. The left hand is grasping the short end and will move towards the body as the right hand moves away to tighten the knot.

from the curled little finger. Hook the back of the right thumb under the right hand thread, extend it so that the thread is angled to the left over the thumb nail (Fig. 43). Encircle the vertical left hand thread with the right index finger. Appose the right index finger to the right thumb, forming a closed ring. Fully supinate the right hand, and the threads will form a crossing lying against the pulp of the right index finger (Fig. 44). Trap the crossing with the thumb. Release the left hand end, fully pronate the right hand, carrying the left hand thread end under the crossing of the threads (Fig. 45). Pick up the short end with your left hand again and bring it towards you, taking the long end away from you with your right hand to tighten the half hitch.

When the short thread is nearest to you, pick up the end with the left hand and hold it vertically. Trap the long thread with the fully flexed middle, ring and little fingers of the right hand, letting the spare thread hang from the little finger. Dip the right index finger under the thread (Fig. 46). Encircle the vertical left hand thread

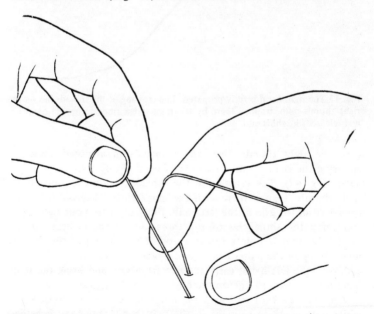

Fig. 46 Two handed knot. The short end is held vertically in the left hand. The right hand holds the long thread, the index finger dipping under it, and about to meet the right thumb which is encircling the short thread.

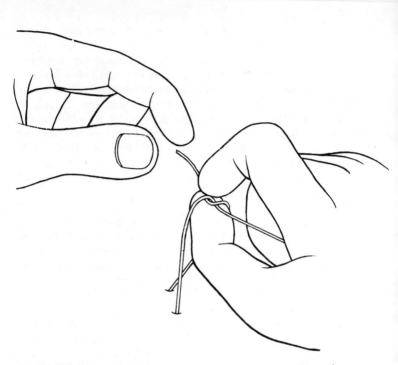

Fig. 47 The right hand is fully pronated. The crossing of the threads lies on the right thumb pulp, trapped there by the right index finger. The left hand has just released the short end.

with the right thumb, from the front. Form a closed circle by apposing the right thumb and index fingers. Fully pronate the right hand (Fig. 47). The crossing of the threads lies on the pulp of the right thumb. Trap it there with the index finger. Release the short thread from the grip of the left hand. Fully supinate your right hand and carry the short end of the thread under the crossing of the threads so that it points towards you. The crossing of the threads now lies upon the pulp of the index finger (Fig. 48). Grasp the short end with the left hand, carry it away from you and bring the right hand towards you to tighten the hitch.

One handed knot tied with the left hand allows you to tie knots while holding an instrument in the right hand. One hand is active, whilst the other, usually holding an instrument, is passive, merely holding one thread whilst the hitches are formed around it. If the

44

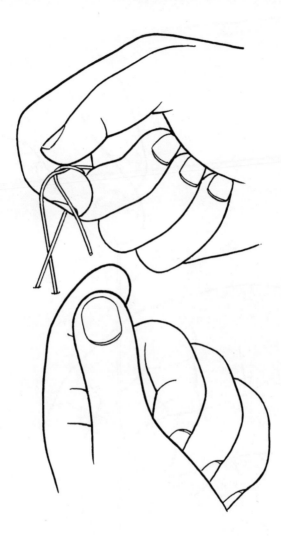

Fig. 48 The right hand is fully supinated carrying the short end under the crossing of the threads which now lies on the pulp of the index finger. The short end will be grasped by the left hand and moved away from the body as the right hand comes towards the body to tighten the knot.

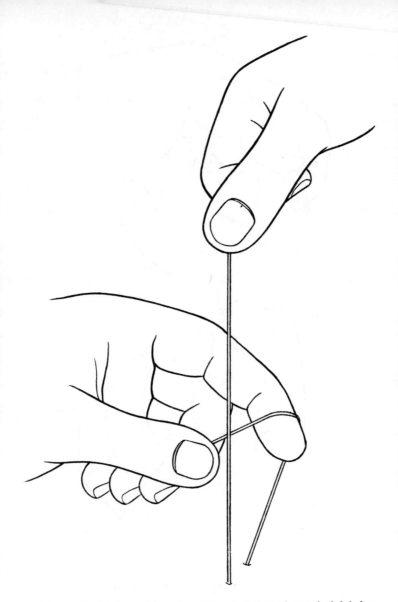

Fig. 49 One handed knot. A crossing of threads is formed over the left index finger.

left hand is holding an instrument, a one handed knot may be formed using the right hand.

If the short end points away from you, pick it up with the left hand between middle finger and thumb, supinating the hand to dip the pulp of the left index finger under the thread to form a loop. Raise the long thread vertically with the right hand so that it lies in contact with the medial aspect of the left index finger. The threads

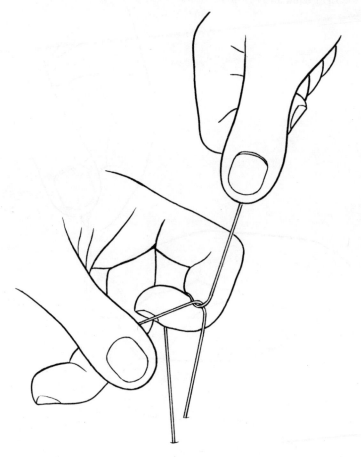

Fig. 50 The left index finger is flexed round the long thread and catches under the short thread.

now form a crossing over this finger (Fig. 49). Flex the tip of the left index finger to curl round the vertically held long thread and catch the short thread with the back of the nail (Fig. 50), carrying a loop downwards and under the crossing of threads that has been formed (Fig. 51). Release the end of the short thread and recapture it with the left hand after it has been drawn under the crossing (Fig. 52). Tighten the hitch by bringing the left hand towards your body and the right hand away from it.

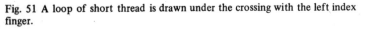

Fig. 51 A loop of short thread is drawn under the crossing with the left index finger.

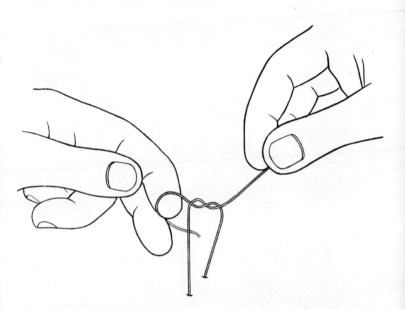

Fig. 52 The short end of thread has been released, drawn under the crossing and recaptured.

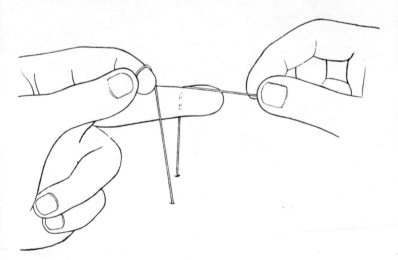

Fig. 53 A crossing of threads is being formed over the left middle finger.

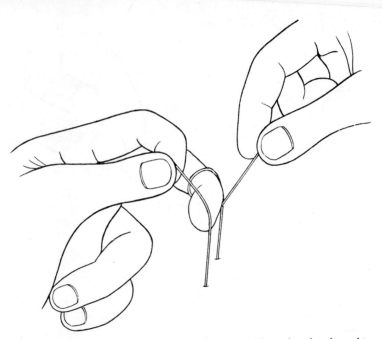

Fig. 54 The left middle finger has curled round the long thread and caught under the short thread.

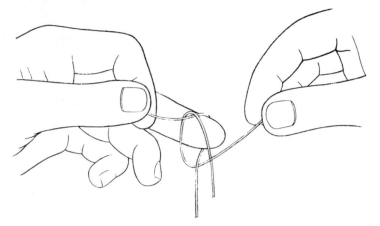

Fig. 55 The left middle finger is extended, drawing a loop of short thread under the crossing of the threads.

If the short end points towards you, pick it up with the left hand between thumb and index finger, supinating the hand and projecting the middle finger so that the short thread crosses its medial aspect. Raise the long thread with the right hand so that it crosses the lateral aspect of the left middle finger (Fig. 53). Flex the left middle finger over the long thread and dip it under the short thread (Fig. 54), extending the finger and pronating the hand to draw a loop of the short thread under the crossing of the threads (Fig. 55). Release the short end of thread and recapture it when it has been drawn under the crossing of the threads (Fig. 56). Tighten the hitch by taking the left hand away from the body and the right hand towards it (Fig. 57).

TYING KNOTS WITH INSTRUMENTS. The fingers or hands may be too large to enter a deep cavity but a needle holder, artery forceps, or dissecting forceps can be used to tie knots within it. When stitching with a needle holder, this may be used to tie the sutures as an alternative to tying one handed knots. Hand tying is wasteful of expensive eyeless needled thread. By using forceps the waste ends can be kept short.

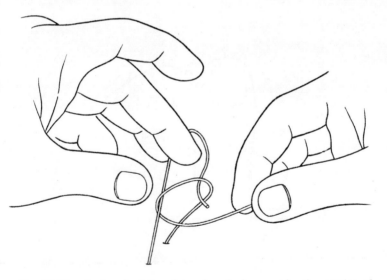

Fig. 56 The short end of thread is released, drawn under the crossing of threads and recaptured with the left hand.

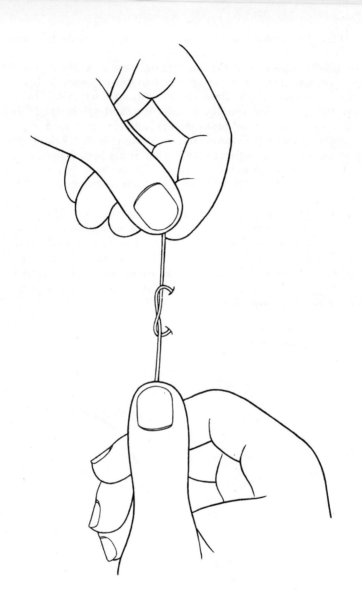

Fig. 57 The half hitch is tightened by carrying the short end away from, the long thread towards, the body.

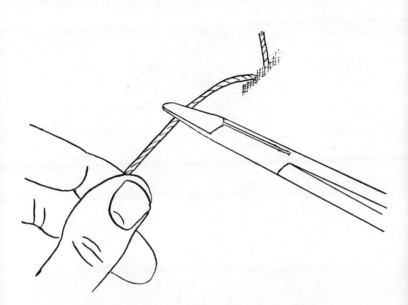

Fig. 58 The forceps blades are laid on the long thread.

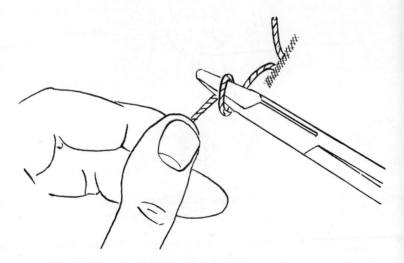

Fig. 59 A turn of long thread has been taken around the forceps blades.

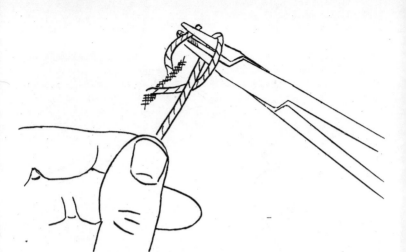

Fig. 60 The forceps grasp the short end through the loop.

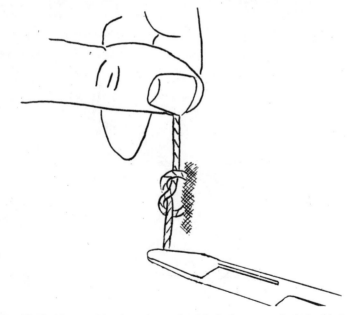

Fig. 61 The short end has been drawn through the loop towards the body, the long end is pushed away, to tighten the hitch.

54

If the short end is farther away, lay the artery forceps (or needle holder) blades on the longer, nearer thread (Fig. 58). Take a turn with the long thread around the forceps (Fig. 59). Grasp the short end with the forceps (Fig. 60) and draw it through the loop in the long end. Tighten the hitch by pushing the long end and drawing the short thread towards you (Fig. 61).

When the short end is towards you, lay the forceps blades on the long thread (Fig. 62). Take a turn with the long thread around the forceps (Fig. 63). Grasp the short end (Fig. 64) and draw it through the loop. Tighten the hitch by drawing the long thread towards you, pushing the short end away (Fig. 65).

Ligatures

A ligature is a binding tied round a structure, most commonly a blood vessel or other duct, usually intended to close the lumen. Ligatures are secured by knotting the ends.

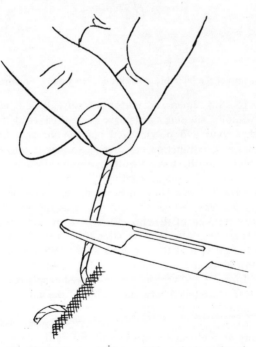

Fig. 62 The forceps blades are laid on the long thread.

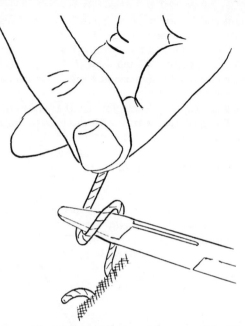

Fig. 63 A turn of the long thread has been taken around the forceps blades.

MATERIALS. Silk, linen and cotton are soft, flexible, can be tied securely without slipping, and have a limited tendency to be reabsorbed. Catgut and polymerized polyglycolic acid threads are absorbed when their function has ceased. Springy stainless steel and monofilament nylon ligatures are difficult to handle and tie securely but they cause minimal tissue reaction.

METHODS. Divided vessels or ducts usually have the ends clamped with artery forceps. While an assistant lifts the handles of the forceps, pass the end of the thread under them, from one hand to the other (Fig. 66). Alternatively stretch the thread between your hands, on the far side of the forceps and get your assistant to reach over the thread to lift the handles of the forceps (Fig. 67). When passing ligatures around vessels or ducts placed deeply in the wound, carry the thread stretched between the tips of the index fingers (Fig. 68). Alternatively use dissecting or artery forceps (Fig. 69), or an aneurysm needle.

To secure an undivided vessel before cutting it, place two artery forceps across it, spaced apart; cut between them and ligate the ends

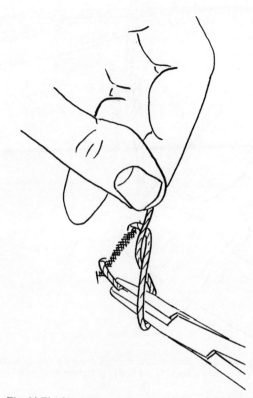

Fig. 64 The forceps grasp the short end through the loop.

(Fig. 70). When the exposed section is short, apply three forceps side by side, remove the middle one, to provide a space in which to divide the vessel (Fig. 71). Alternatively the duct or vessel may first be doubly ligated in continuity by passing the thread with dissecting forceps, curved artery forceps, or with an aneurysm needle (Fig. 72). Two ligatures are usually tied and the structure is then cut between them. To separate the ligatures tie one and pass the uncut thread to an assistant to apply traction, while passing and tying the next ligature at the opposite extremity of the structure. A second method is to place an artery forceps across the middle of the exposed portion and tie ligatures on either side of it, then remove the artery forceps and divide the segment crushed by the forceps blades.

SAFETY. Use suitable material for the intended purpose and ensure

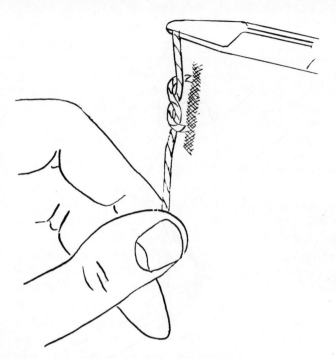

Fig. 65 The short end has been drawn through the loop and is pushed away while the long end is drawn towards the body, to tighten the hitch.

that you have a sufficient length of the correct thread. Too strong thread may cut right through the structure; too weak material may break. Never tie a ligature too near the cut end of a vessel or duct, but leave a projection so that the ligature cannot slide off the end (Fig. 73). Make sure you have only the intended structure encircled in the ligature. Especially take care to avoid tying in the tip of artery forceps; when they are moved, the ligature will be pulled off.

When tying a ligature next to an artery forceps, instruct the assistant to relax the grip of the forceps just as the circle of thread tightens, otherwise the constricting effect of the ligature is lost. The forceps must not be removed completely until the ligature is secure. In hazardous situations have the assistant retighten the clamp until ordered to remove it. Tie a second ligature over the first or near it, as an added precaution.

Transfixion suture prevents the ligature slipping off the end of a

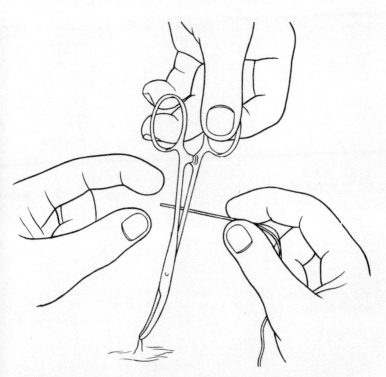

Fig. 66 The handles of the artery forceps have been raised by an assistant as a ligature is passed under them.

divided structure. Pierce the structure with the ligature thread mounted on a needle. Encircle half the circumference and tie a half hitch, then encircle the whole structure and tie a complete knot (Fig. 74).

Never rely upon a ligature to close a wide-bore or rigid tube. Instead, flatten the end and close it with a row of sutures. The end of a large but deformable tube may be ligated and then invaginated within a purse-string suture applied proximal to the ligature (Fig. 75).

When tying a ligature around a thick structure, 'bed' it down by repeatedly pulling, but not jerking, the threads after tying the first half hitch (Fig. 76). If the half hitch slips, tie a surgeon's knot initially.

Do not let your assistant undo all your safety precautions by cutting the threads too short.

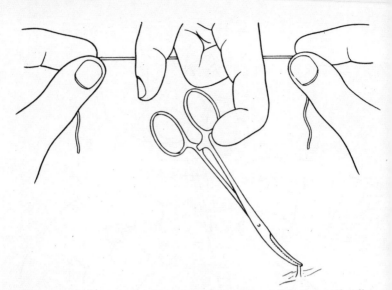

Fig. 67 The stretched thread has been advanced beyond the forceps handles and the assistant is about to lift the handles over the thread.

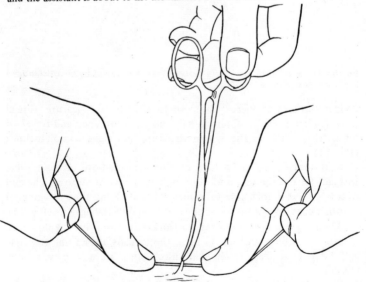

Fig. 68 The ligature thread stretched between the index finger tips is carried under the projecting tips of an artery forceps.

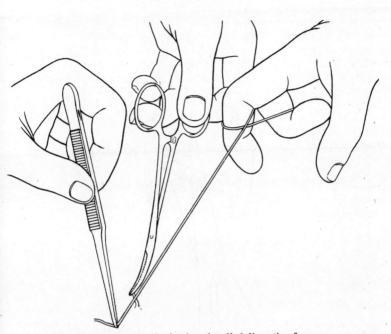

Fig. 69 Ligature passed using long handled dissecting forceps.

LENGTH OF LIGATURES. When the knot must be tied in the depths of a cavity, 30 cm lengths of thread are ideal. This length may be used to tie several ligatures at the surface. Feed the thread through the fingers of the right hand. Some operators attach a bobbin of ligature thread to their wrist, or hold an egg-shaped ligature container in the palm of the hand when tying multiple ligatures.

Stitching

Versatile thread stitches are peerless for joining together tissues that can be pierced with a needle, in spite of ingenious attempts to supersede them with metal clips, and adhesives. Threads are carried by the needle through the tissues and fixed by knotting them.

If two portions are to be joined the stitch is carried through one, then the other, and the ends of thread are joined. A portion of tissue may be deliberately constricted to stop or prevent bleeding by using a stitch. A stitch offers a temorary grip of tissue and the thread ends may be left long in order to apply gentle traction. A tied stitch of

61

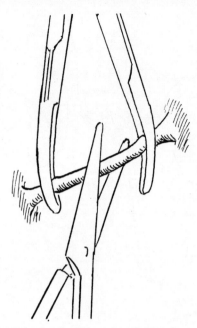

Fig. 70 The vessel is doubly clamped and divided between the forceps.

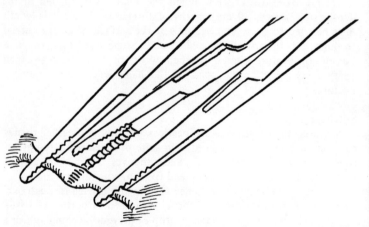

Fig. 71 Three artery forceps are applied side by side across the vessel. The centre forceps are removed, leaving a space to divide the vessel.

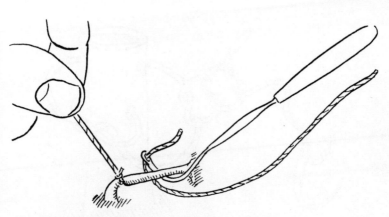

Fig. 72 Passing ligatures around an undivided vessel using an aneurysm needle. One ligature has been passed, tied, the end left long and traction is applied to it. The second ligature is passed and tied at the other end of the exposed segment of vessel. The vessel will be divided between the ligatures.

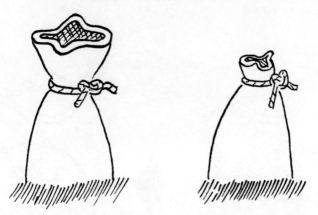

Fig. 73 The ligature on the left is safe and will not slip off. The ligature on the right is too near the end of the vessel and is likely to slip off.

striking coloured thread is a useful marker to aid subsequent identification of a tissue. A ligature can be secured against slipping by inserting a stitch before tying it.

Weak areas may be strengthened by inserting a darn. The thread is run back and forth between stitch holes without being pulled tight enough to draw the holes together.

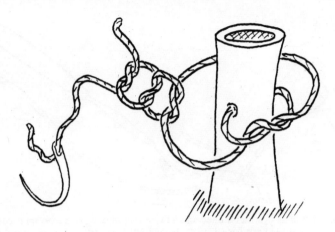

Fig. 74 Transfixion suture ligature. The needled thread has been taken through the structure, a half hitch is tied, then the whole structure is encircled and a complete knot is tied.

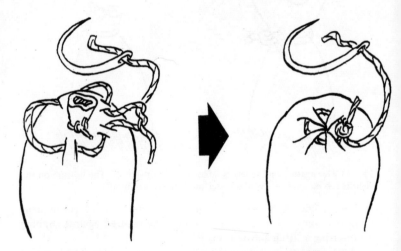

Fig. 75 On the left a ligature has been tied to close the end of a large duct. On the right the closed end has been invaginated with a purse-string suture.

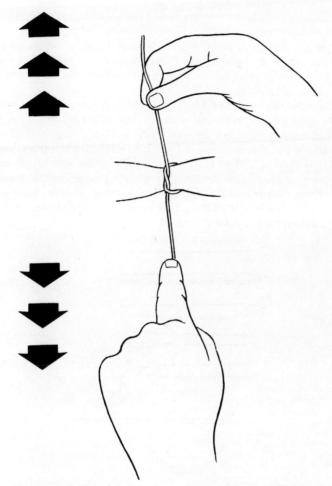

Fig. 76 'Bed' down a ligature around a thick structure by tightening the first half hitch several times.

NEEDLES (Fig. 77). Fragile tissue can be pierced with round-bodied needles similar to those used for sewing cloth, and they produce minimal damage. Fibrous tissues are resistant and cutting needles, with triangular or flat cross-sections, must be used.

Needle eyes are usually similar to those of needles employed for sewing cloth. In order to minimize damage from stitching, the

65

needles may be swaged on to the thread and are often called 'eyeless' or 'atraumatic' needles.

Needles may be straight, when the track through the tissues is straight or can be straightened. Curved needles are used when the track the needle must follow is curved. The curve may or may not form an arc of a circle.

STITCHING WITH A STRAIGHT NEEDLE. A straight needle held in the hand is the most natural means of introducing stitches.

A straight needle can be used only when the needle track is straight or the tissues can be deformed to straighten the track, and provided there is a clear exit for the needle. Many soft tissues are amenable to temporary deformation while a straight needle transfixes them. The two edges of a skin incision may be lifted together and everted while a straight cutting needle is passed through both edges. Bowel may be similarly sutured.

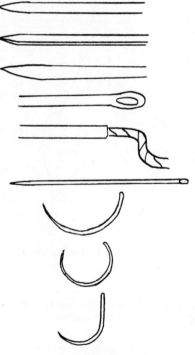

Fig. 77 Needles.

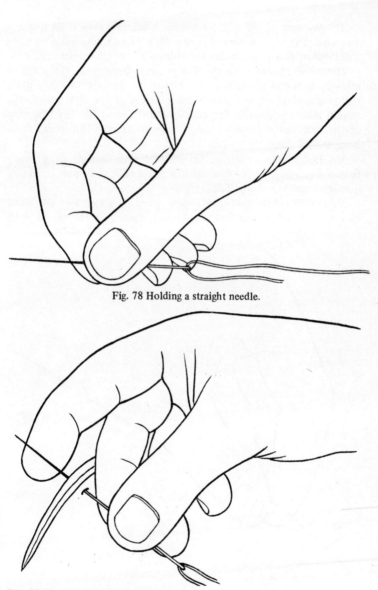

Fig. 78 Holding a straight needle.

Fig. 79 The needle is controlled by pressure of the thumb against the middle and ring fingers, releasing the index finger to lift the emerging point.

Do not despise the straight needle. Used with skill, it is rapid and effective. Do not use thread longer than 40–45 cm. Make sure the short end of thread protrudes for at least 5 cm beyond the eye.

Hold the needle with the point away from you, the hand at midway between pronation and supination, the shaft resting upon the pulps of the index and middle fingers of the right hand, the thumb pulp compressing the needle against them (Fig. 78). The pulp of the ring finger presses upon the eye to prevent the thread from being pulled out.

Manipulate the tissues to be stitched with the left hand, using fingers or dissecting forceps, so that the needle may pass correctly through them in a straight line.

You may stitch with the needle pointing away and the hand partially supinated. For fast and easy stitching grip the needle with

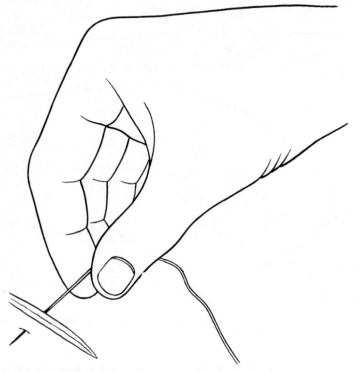

Fig. 80 Stitching with the needle pointing towards you.

thumb opposing the middle and ring fingers, reserving the index finger to lift the emerging pointed end (Fig. 79). The pressure of the thumb is then transferred to grip the emerging needle against the index finger pulp, and draw it through.

Alternatively you may partially pronate the hand and sew with the point towards you (Fig. 80), the thumb and index fingers transferring to the emerging section of needle to draw it through.

When a thick segment of tissue is transfixed, the grip may need to be transferred nearer the needle eye to give it a second thrust.

The left hand arranges and steadies the tissues directly or with dissecting forceps. Alternatively it may 'follow-up' during continuous suturing, keeping the emerging thread at the correct tension and incidentally steadying the tissues in this way for the next stitch (Fig. 81). The left ring finger helps to steady the tissues against the

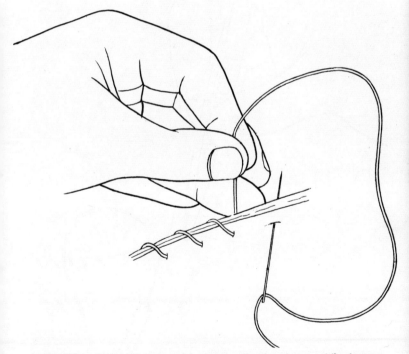

Fig. 81 The left hand 'follows-up' by holding the thread taut, while the next stitch is inserted. Notice the left ring finger tip steadies the tissues against the thrust of the needle.

thrust of the needle. In some situations the left hand, either directly or with dissecting forceps, may catch the emerging needle point to draw it through or steady it while transferring the grip of the right hand.

Some surgeons prefer to sew from right to left, others prefer left to right. The choice often depends upon the difficulty of apposing the tissues, and therefore the demands made upon the left hand to hold them together while inserting the stitches. If this is difficult, it is usually preferable to work towards the left hand, that is, from right to left (Fig. 82).

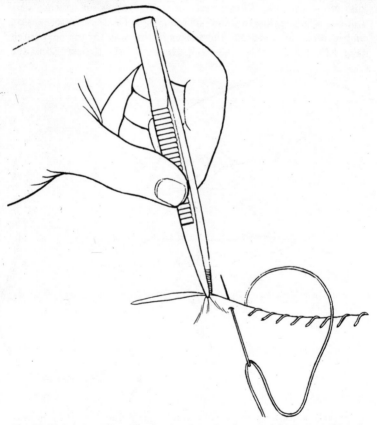

Fig. 82 The tissues are apposed using dissecting forceps held in the left hand, while sewing from right to left.

STITCHING WITH A CURVED NEEDLE. Whenever the tissues cannot be moulded to allow the passage of a straight needle, use a curved needle. This can be driven in along a curved path so that the tip emerges at a distance from the point of entry.

Hand-held needles can suitably be used when large 'bites' of tissue must be taken. Hold the needle between thumb and the lateral pulp of the middle finger, eye on the right point on the left, both pointing towards you, convexity away from you, steadied by the pulp of your index finger (Fig. 83). Try to stitch towards yourself, driving the needle by flexing the wrist. Allow it to follow its natural path. When the point emerges, draw it out along the same curved path. Press the pulp of the ring finger against the eye of the needle to trap the thread while drawing the stitch taut. Alternatively grasp the needle against the palm using the medial fingers, while drawing the stitch taut using thumb and index finger.

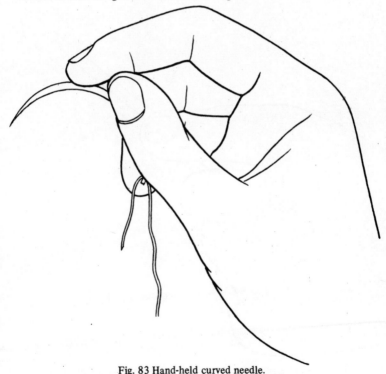

Fig. 83 Hand-held curved needle.

Instrument-held needles that are too small to be manipulated with the hand are mounted in the jaws of a needle holder, point to the left, eye to the right, both pointing upwards, convexity down. The shank is gripped just to the eye side of the midpoint. The eye is a weak point of the needle and must not be grasped by the jaws of the needle holder.

Whenever possible insert the needle from right to left, or towards you, starting with the hand fully pronated (Fig. 84). The needle points downwards, to be driven through the tissues by supinating the wrist (Fig. 85). Grasp the emerging needle with fingers or forceps to

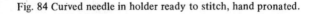

Fig. 84 Curved needle in holder ready to stitch, hand pronated.

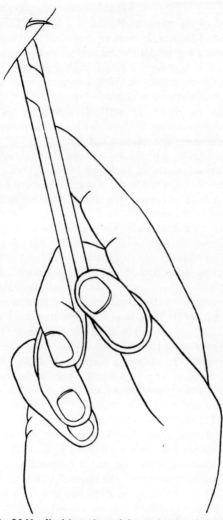

Fig. 85 Needle driven through by supinating the wrist.

draw it through in the line of its curve. Regrasp the needle correctly in the needle holder, ready for the next stitch, as the thread is drawn taut. In difficult situations it may be preferable merely to steady the emerging needle, unclamp the needle holder from the shank of the needle and use it to grasp the pointed end to draw it through. Take care not to grasp the point itself, which will quite likely break off, leaving the rest of the needle elusively buried in the tissues. Draw the needle out along a curved path while supinating the wrist.

Occasionally it is necessary to stitch by passing the needle from right to left or away from you. This is very much more difficult. In some awkward situations, a change of posture may allow familiar movements to be made. In difficult situations take each step carefully; rough handling will end with a broken or bent needle, troublesome bleeding, and insecure stitching.

Atraumatic needles pass easily through the tissues, reducing the drag as the thread is drawn through. Never tighten the stitch by pulling on the needle, always grasp the thread between the needle and the stitch hole, otherwise the thread will be pulled from the tubular channel of the needle.

CONTROL OF THE THREAD. Keep spare thread looped well clear so that it does not become entangled. Do not use too long a thread, but on the other hand do not struggle with too short a thread.

When stitching with stiff thread such as stainless steel wire, or monofilamentous nylon, ensure that your assistant follows it through as you draw on the thread, to prevent it from kinking.

INTERRUPTED STITCHES have the advantage that when used in series the failure of one stitch does not necessarily prejudice the others. The types of stitch are copied from, and therefore named after, ancient methods of sewing cloth or skins (Fig. 86), although the names of pioneers who popularized their use in surgery is often attached. Each stitch is secured with a knot, although exceptionally the ends may be trapped by clamping on a lead button.

CONTINUOUS STITCHES have the advantage of being quick to insert and of having fewer knots, which are the weak points of stitches. If a simple over and over stitch is used, the tissue is not encircled and rendered ischaemic, but is traversed by a spiral thread which can adjust to, and spread, the tension. Varieties of continuous stitches (Fig. 87) may be used, some incorporating a locking loop that prevents slipping of tissues drawn together under tension, as stitching proceeds. Make sure the thread 'beds down' correctly as each stitch is tightened. If it tends to twist upon itself, gently lift the loop using a finger or forceps, until it is almost tight.

At the beginning of the run the first stitch is taken, the thread is partly pulled through, and the end is captured and tied to the long emerging thread. At the end of a run of continuous stitching the short end may be grasped before the last stitch is inserted and tied to

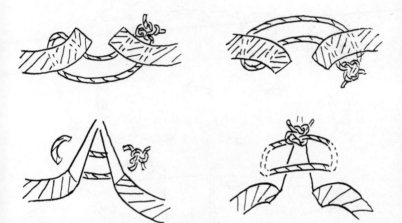

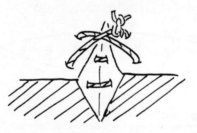

Fig. 86 Interrupted stitches. Top; simple interrupted. Second line, longitudinal mattress, everting on the left inverting on the right. Third line; horizontal mattress, everting on the left, inverting on the right. Bottom; 'X' stitch.

the loop that is threaded on the needle. If an eyeless needle is used, the loop before the last stitch is tied to the end. If the thread is insufficiently long to complete the stitch it is usually tied off, the next stitch is tied and run on. If the end of the first stitch is short, or if it has broken, the new stitch may be inserted and tied, and the

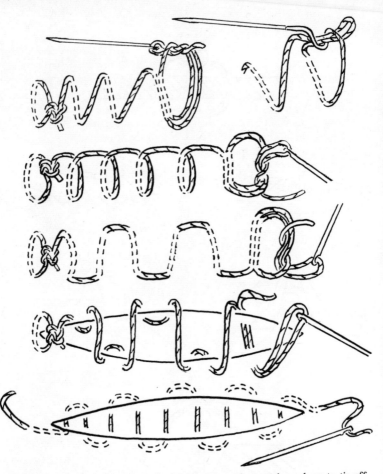

Fig. 87 Continuous stitches. Top; simple over and over; shows how to tie off the thread; on the left with an ordinary needle, on the right with an eyeless needle. Second line, locking or blanket stitch. Third line, everting mattress. Fourth line, inverting mattress or Connell stitch. Bottom; subcuticular.

short end of the first thread is then tied to the end of the new thread.

STITCHING IN DIFFERENT TISSUES requires different techniques and materials.

Skin must be brought into accurate apposition, without excessive tension and without the interposition of subcutaneous fat, hairs, suture material or blood clot. The stitches must be tied just tight enough to appose the edges, taking into account the oedema that will occur during the next few days. The outer layers of skin which are dead and cornified must not be apposed by inverting the skin edges; rather the edges should be slightly everted to bring together the living deeper layers. This is achieved by everting the edges before inserting the needle, or by using a mattress suture which has an everting action. The edges of an incision should be stitched together in their original position. This may not be possible in angulated wounds or during plastic procedures. Perfect apposition is aided in a straight wound if it is stretched lengthways by an assistant drawing apart the ends using skin hooks, tissue forceps, or by traction on the ends of the stitches.

Skin is usually stitched using fine non-absorbable material such as silk, cotton or nylon which will be removed when the edges are sufficiently adherent; removal is facilitated if the thread is dyed to contrast with skin colour. Eyeless needles reduce damage. The skin should not be grasped or crushed with heavy forceps. In order to achieve the best cosmetic results, skin stitches are made to extend as little as possible from the wound edges, and they are removed as early as possible—after two or three days in certain situations.

Small metal clips may also be used to close skin wounds. By means of special forceps they are clamped across the wound so small points at each end grip the skin to draw together and evert the edges. The clips are subsequently removed by opening them out to withdraw the points using special forceps. Adherent strips of material may be applied across wound edges to appose them while healing takes place. They avoid the need to puncture the skin.

Bowel is usually stitched using catgut that will be absorbed. It is mounted on eyeless needles, and is usually inserted as a continuous stitch. The strongest part of the bowel wall is the collagenous submucosa and this is best caught in a stitch that traverses all the coats of the bowel. Since the mucosa may be extruded between stitches it is traditional to invert the bowel wall, apposing the serosal surfaces that rapidly form a sealed closure. The bowel may be held inverted while inserting the stitches, or mattress stitches may be so placed that they draw together the outer surfaces of the bowel wall. The all-coats stitch is usually reinforced by a second layer of stitches, picking up the serosa and underlying muscle, that improve the apposition of the peritoneal surfaces. This may be a catgut or non-absorbable stitch. The bowel must not be encircled with a tight,

77

continuous, non-absorbable stitch or the lumen may be obstructed.

Blood vessels must be sutured to present the smoothest possible surface to the flow of blood, since irregularity provokes clot deposition with subsequent occlusion of the lumen. Exceptionally fine thread, swaged on fine eyeless needles, dyed black to give it colour contrast, is inserted as an over and over stitch while everting the vessel edges to bring together the smooth endothelial linings. Eversion may be encouraged by inserting suitable mattress stitches.

Fascia is sutured using absorbable or non-absorbable thread mounted on strong cutting-edged needles. The direction of the fascial fibres must be considered; if they run at right angles to the edges of the wound, simple stitches would tend to cut out, so horizontal mattress sutures are usually preferable (Fig. 88). If the fibres are predominantly parallel to the edges of the wound, stitches should not all be inserted at the same distance from the edges, or they may detach a strip of parallel fibrous bundles (Fig. 89).

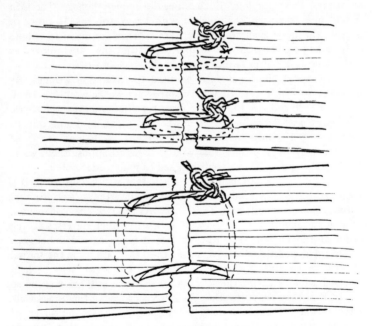

Fig. 88 Stitching fascia with fibres at right angles to edges. Simple stitches (above) tend to cut out. Horizontal mattress sutures (below) hold better.

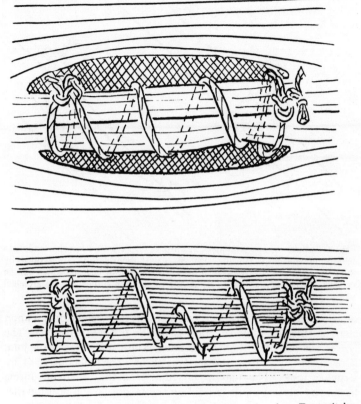

Fig. 89 Stitching fascia with fibres running parallel to the edges. Top: stitches inserted all at the same distance from the edges tend to drag away a strip of fascia. Bottom: stitches hold better if they are inserted at varying distances from the edges.

Tendons consist of parallel fibres relatively poorly bound together, so that simple stitches would rapidly cut out under the powerful tractive forces. Additionally the tendon may glide in a smooth sheath and would be impeded by irregularities along its length. Whenever possible the tendon is therefore criss-crossed with stitches on each side of the join to spread the traction (Fig. 90). Fine, strong, non-absorbable suture material, such as stainless steel wire is inserted on eyeless needles. When smooth action is important, the thread is looped and the bight is caught and anchored to the

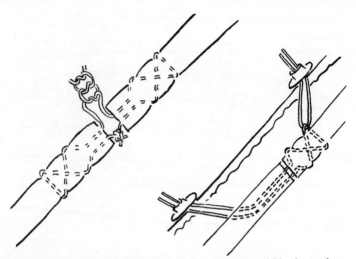

Fig. 90 Sutures joining tendons. The stitches criss-cross within the tendon to achieve greater grip. On the right is a withdrawable stitch described by Bunnell. The ends are trapped at skin level with lead buttons which can be detached. The bight can then be drawn to the skin surface by the attached loop.

surface so that when healing is complete the loop can be drawn upon and the thread withdrawn, thus removing all foreign material. The largest possible area of tendon is brought into apposition at the join, if necessary by cutting the surfaces to be joined obliquely, or by stepping them. The tension is reduced to the minimum during healing by placing joints crossed by the tendon in the position that will relax it.

Nerves. Exact apposition of divided nerves is essential if a satisfactory result is hoped for following repair. Misalignment prevents nerve fibres from reaching the correct end-organs. Stitches are placed in the perineurium or outer sheath using the finest material such as silk or stainless steel mounted on eyeless needles.

Muscles. Relaxed skeletal muscle is difficult to sew if it has been divided across the fibres, since stitches cut out. Unless the muscle can be relaxed until the scar is strong, the stitches easily tear out. Absorbable catgut sutures are usually inserted as mattress stitches. When the muscle fibres run parallel to the suture line, do not overtighten the simple catgut stitches apposing the edges or the fibres will be constricted, become fibrous, and lose their contractility.

Bone. Soft tissues can be attached to bone by stitching them to the periosteum or ligaments using chromicized catgut mounted on heavy needles with triangular (trocar) points. Alternatively the bone may be drilled and stitches are then passed through the holes. Wire sutures may be passed through drill holes, and bone pieces may also be screwed together or joined by metal plates. The retained metal is of special material that will not provoke a reaction in the tissues.

Fat. Areolar connective tissue containing fat does not hold stitches well. It is therefore useless to sew it with heavy gauge thread. Fine minimally chromicized catgut is sufficiently strong and will soon be absorbed.

VARIATION IN TECHNIQUES. Successful operators often believe that the type of materials, needles, or stitches they use are the secret of their success. They are too modest since success comes from carrying out the right procedure correctly. Provided stitching is carried out with the minimum of trauma, with the best apposition of tissues, with suitable material, then the size and shape of the needle, selection of thread, and types of stitch, are personal matters.

Learn the orthodox techniques and those used by masters. Follow them until you have attained self-confidence, then adapt their techniques to suit yourself. Do not, however, change for its own sake. Established techniques are accepted generally because they are the ones that most people have come to trust.

Chapter 4

HANDLING DUCTS

Ducts subserve many functions in the body. They may be mere conduits for blood and other fluids, the vis a tergo (push from behind) being supplied by a pump. Some tubes, such as bowel, have intrinsic peristalsis that transports the contents along. Some ducts and vessels have specialized segments acting as valves, metering the flow through them. Substances may be added to the contents, and absorbed actively or passively from the fluid as it passes along the tube. Peripheral nerves may be considered as cabled nerve ducts. Ducts may be created surgically, or result from disease (sinuses or fistulas). The mechanical qualities of the various ducts imposes varying techniques when dissecting, repairing, opening, closing or uniting them.

Location

Some ducts, such as the bowel, lie free while others are buried in connective tissues. The ability to find and recognize a duct is improved by becoming familiar with its feel and appearance. The pulsations of an artery may be palpable, as may the distinctive cartilagenous rings of the trachea and major bronchi. The contents may be visible, such as blood within a thin-walled blood vessel, which appears blue. The ureter has a characteristic vermiculating peristaltic movement. Some ducts can be traced from their origin such as breast ducts, the ureters and urethra, and sinuses or fistulas resulting from disease or produced deliberately, that open upon the surface. The track can be located by inserting a probe or a catheter, and if the track is very convoluted, by filling it with distinctive dye. Lymphatic vessels take up Vital Blue Dye that has been injected into the surrounding tissues, and then become easily visible. Ducts may be located radiologically after injecting radio-opaque media into them. Certain radio-opaque substances administered orally or parenterally are excreted into ducts and may be displayed on X-ray films.

When seeking a duct lying in homogeneous tissue, always cut in the expected line of the duct rather than at right angles to it, to avoid inadvertently transecting the duct.

Display

If a long segment of duct must be dissected out in order to display it, take care to preserve any tributaries, branches, nerves or vessels. When displaying major blood vessels, first ensure before embarking upon a hazardous dissection, that you are able to control bleeding if the vessel is inadvertently opened. Place an open non-crushing clamp across it, encircle it with a tape that can be tightened, or get an assistant to hold the vessel between finger and thumb, ready to compress it.

The dissection should be carried out in a manner that will not damage the structure to be displayed. Fragile overlying connective tissue may be split by pushing the rounded tips of closed dissecting forceps blades alongside the duct. If it is necessary to cut the overlying tissues protect a vulnerable duct by inserting fine non-toothed forceps superficial to the duct along its track and cut into the groove between the blades of the forceps using a scalpel or scissors (Fig. 91).

Blunt-nosed haemostatic forceps make good dissecting instruments when freeing firm ducts such as blood vessels. The closed

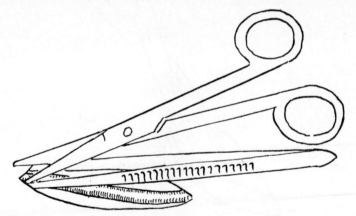

Fig. 91 Displaying a vessel by placing dissecting forceps superficial to it and cutting the overlying tissues between the forceps blades.

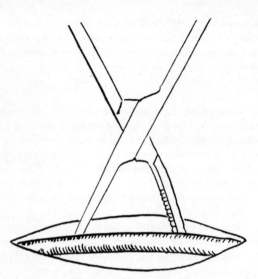

Fig. 92 Displaying a vessel using haemostatic forceps opened parallel to the vessel.

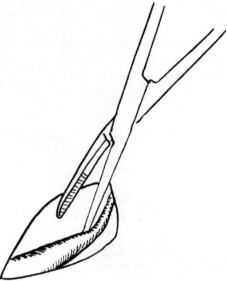

Fig. 93 Displaying a vessel using haemostatic forceps opened at right angles to the vessel.

blades are insinuated alongside the vessel and the forceps are then gently opened. Try opening the blades parallel to the vessel (Fig. 92) or alternatively at right angles to it (Fig. 93).

Percutaneous cannulation

Superficial veins that can be seen and arteries that can be palpated, may be cannulated without first displaying them direct. Certain hidden ducts and vessels may be cannulated blindly, such as dilated intrahepatic bile ducts, splenic blood vessels, and hollow spaces distended with fluid such as the urinary bladder, heart chambers, cerebral ventricles, and pathological collections such as effusions, cysts, haematomas, and abscesses (Fig. 94).

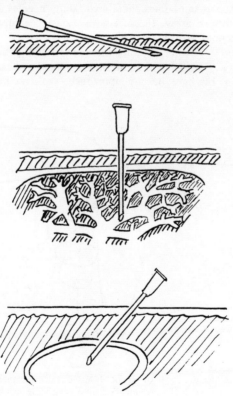

Fig. 94 Cannulating at top a superficial vessel, at centre labyrinthine vessels in an organ, at bottom a cavity.

Vessels, ducts and spaces are most easily entered when they are distended with fluid. Veins may be dilated by making the part dependent, by applying warmth and by congesting them using pressure applied proximally with a finger or constricting cuff. Veins may be better seen if obscuring skin hair is shaved off.

Veins and arteries slip easily from beneath the needle and should be fixed and straightened by stretching them with the overlying skin. In the case of peripheral vessels this can easily be achieved by finger or thumb pressure and by moving the nearby joints (Fig. 95).

HOLLOW NEEDLES are inserted alone, or as pilots for other cannulae. As a rule they are first attached to a syringe to collect fluid, and to form a closed system. They are bevelled to produce a cutting edge and this is sometimes chamfered. Many needles are used once only and thrown away. If a needle is used repeatedly, ensure that the point is not distorted or turned over.

Venepuncture. When entering a fragile vein first puncture the skin to one side, so preventing unintentional damage to the vein. When the whole of the bevel lies subcutaneously, angle the needle to enter

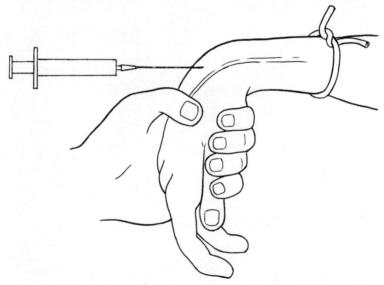

Fig. 95 The needle is about to be inserted into a superficial vein by percutaneous puncture. To distend the vein a congesting cuff has been placed around the forearm. To fix the vein the thumb has been placed over the distal part, and to straighten it and fix it, the subject's wrist has been flexed.

the vein. Blood will now flow into the syringe, or may be aspirated into it. Advance the needle into the vein. From time to time stop the advance, raise the point of the needle to see if it lifts the superficial vein wall, confirming that it remains within the lumen. When the needle is advanced sufficiently, confirm that it lies within the vein by aspirating a little blood. Leave some of the shank outside the skin as a safeguard against the needle breaking at the neck between shank and syringe connection. Unless blood is to be aspirated, release the proximal congesting cuff. When attempting to puncture thick-walled veins that tend to slip away from the needle, try to start the venepuncture at the junction of tributaries where the vein tends to be relatively fixed (Fig. 96). When cannulating fragile thin-walled veins do not over congest them or they rupture as soon as they are punctured.

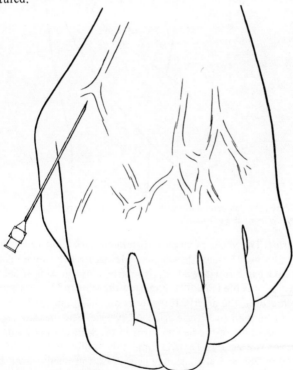

Fig. 96 The needle is about to enter a superficial vein at the junction of tributaries where the draining vessel is relatively fixed.

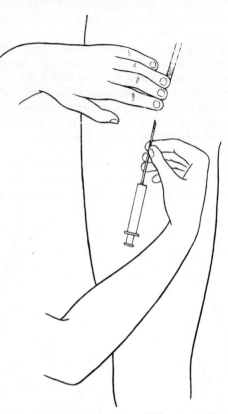

Fig. 97 Percutaneous cannulation of an artery. The artery is located and fixed with the fingers of the left hand.

Arteries. The vessel is already distended with fluid unless it is in spasm. The needle may slip to one side because the vessel is freely mobile and has a tough wall. Fix the artery by pressing it against a firm base if possible (Fig. 97). Puncture the skin and lay the point of the needle over the artery. Enter it at an angle and small spurts of blood can be seen to fill the attached syringe. The pressure required to push the point of the needle through the wall is usually sufficient to collapse the artery. To overcome this, deliberately transfix the artery (Fig. 98) and then slowly withdraw the needle until blood spurts back into the syringe. Advance the needle point gently along the lumen, avoiding damage to the lining and artery wall.

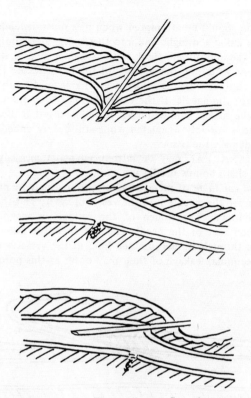

Fig. 98 Cannulating an artery. The needle transfixes the artery at the top, is gradually withdrawn in the centre, and advanced within the lumen at the bottom.

Labyrinthine vessels within an organ may be cannulated by percutaneous needle puncture. The blood vessels of the spleen and dilated intrahepatic bile ducts are entered through the skin using needles. To minimize the damage, relative movement between skin and the organ is stopped by preventing respiration while the needle is in place. The organ is entered deeply by a thrust of the needle in a straight line through the skin and intervening tissues. It is then withdrawn slowly while gentle suction is applied, until blood or fluid is aspirated indicating that the tip of the needle lies within the appropriate vessel.

Cavities may be recognizable anatomical spaces or artificial spaces delineated by physical signs or radiography. If a cavity varies in size,

89

cannulation should be attempted when it is most distended. Thrust the needle along a straight line into the cavity, and confirm this by aspirating the appropriate fluid. If fluid cannot be aspirated, do not immediately withdraw the needle but rotate it, in case the bevel is sealed by contact with the cavity wall. If this fails, gently withdraw and advance the needle. If the cavity has not been entered, do not angulate the needle but withdraw it and re-insert it along a fresh track; if it is forcibly angulated while still deeply imbedded it will break, or damage the tissues.

BLUNT CANNULAE may be introduced percutaneously (Fig. 99) utilizing a sharp hollow needle as a guide.

Internal cannulae of metal or plastic tubing may be passed along the lumen of the needle into the vessel or cavity and the needle is then withdrawn. The lumen of the cannula is inevitably much smaller than that of the needle and can therefore take only slow flow rates through it. Because the hole in the vessel wall is larger than the cannula, leakage of fluid may occur at this point after the

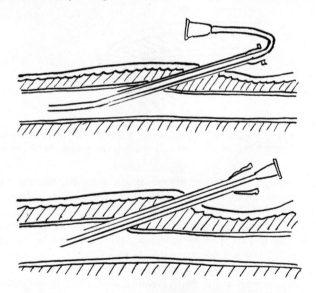

Fig. 99 Inserting blunt cannulae percutaneously using a sharp needle as a pilot. The upper diagram shows a cannula passed through the lumen of the needle. The lower diagram shows the cannula fitted closely to the outside of the needle.

needle is withdrawn. If the cannula has an expanded connector for a syringe, the needle cannot be removed. The needle point may pierce a plastic cannula, causing a fluid leak. This has been ingeniously overcome by the development of needles that are split along their length and can be separated longitudinally into two halves, and so removed, after withdrawing them from the skin.

External cannulae. A metal or plastic cylinder that fits closely to the outside of the needle has the outstanding advantage of having a lumen wider than the needle. Plastic tubing that is heated and drawn

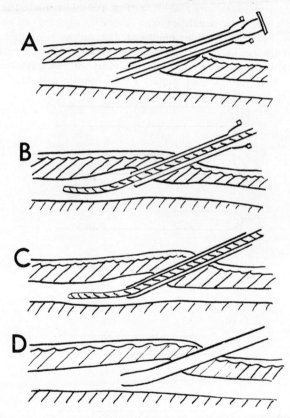

Fig. 100 Seldinger's guide wire technique. At A the vessel is cannulated. The needle is withdrawn and replaced at B with the guide wire. The cannula is withdrawn and replaced at C by the plastic catheter. At D the guide wire is removed.

out into a thinner segment may be cut off and snugly fitted over the needle. The needle point projects beyond the tip of the cannula. The overlying skin should be nicked to prevent it from hindering the passage of the cannula. Insert the needle into the vessel or cavity, aspirate fluid to confirm this, and then advance it. Firmly but controllably overcome the resistance to the passage of the cannula tip by the vessel or cavity wall. Once the cannula has entered the lumen, it may be advanced, leaving the needle behind, or the needle may be withdrawn, leaving the cannula within the lumen.

Seldinger's guide wire technique (Fig. 100). Cannulate the vessel with a wide bore needle or with a needle carrying an external cannula. Pass the flexible, blunt-ended, stainless steel guide wire through the needle or cannula and withdraw the needle or cannula, meanwhile compressing the point of entry of the guide wire to prevent extraversation of blood. Pass a plastic catheter, with a

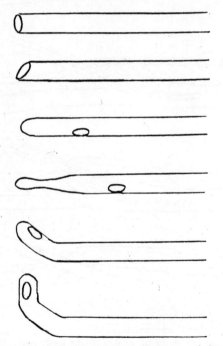

Fig. 101 Catheter tips. From above downwards: open end, flute tip, round end with side hole, olivary tip, coudé and bicoudé.

leading edge shaped to fit the guide wire closely, over the wire and advance it into the lumen. When the resistance of the vessel wall is felt, grasp the catheter and wire together, withdraw them slightly, then advance them smoothly together to carry the catheter into the lumen. Withdraw the guide wire.

Direct cannulation

Vessels, ducts, and cavities may be cannulated directly either because they communicate with the surface, or because though they lie deeply they have been displayed.

Metal, gum-elastic, rubber, or plastic catheters may be used with plain open ends, oblique ends, closed ends with side holes, and with straight or curved tips (Fig. 101). Choose one of the correct size and shape that will slip easily in contact with the lining of the vessel or duct. The largest size that will pass easily is usually preferable to allow the maximum flow rate, and the least risk of blockage.

INSERTION. A cannula may be passed into the end of an open duct such as the urethra, an external sinus or fistula, or an exposed, transected internal duct. Steady the ends of the duct, if necessary, with traction stitches or tissue-holding forceps.

Intact ducts and vessels may be cannulated through longitudinal or transverse incisions in the wall. If the cannula is intended to fill the lumen of the vessel, tie off the vessel proximal to the direction

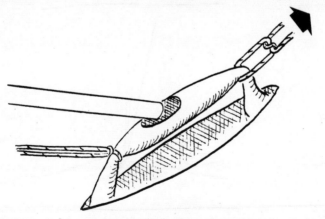

Fig. 102 The duct has been tied off on the left and traction is exerted with the ligature thread. On the right a ligature is passed but not tightened, and drawn to the right, steadying the duct while the cannula is inserted.

93

the catheter will take, and place a second ligature, tied with a half hitch but not tightened, around the part of the vessel that will receive the cannula. Stretch the vessel between these two ligatures to steady it while introducing the tip of the cannula (Fig. 102). When the cannula is in place, secure it by tightening the loose ligature and completing the knot.

Incise fine ducts after lifting a small portion of the wall with fine forceps and using obliquely held scissors, cutting in the direction that the cannula will take, to cut a 'V' flap (Fig. 103). Hold up the

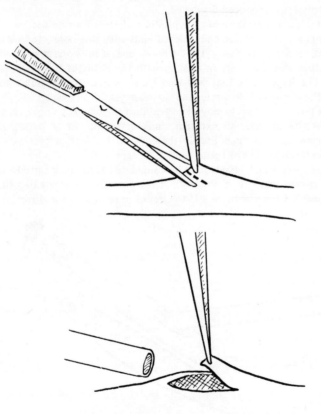

Fig. 103 The upper diagram shows the duct being opened obliquely to produce a 'V' flap. In the lower diagram the flap is raised and the cannula is about to be inserted.

flap with the forceps and slip the tip of the cannula underneath it to enter the lumen.

Very fine ducts such as lymphatic vessels may be cannulated using fine, sharp, hollow needles. Work in good light, wear magnifying spectacles if necessary, and steady your hands against a firm base. Try not to puncture the vessel until the needle enters, or the fluid leaks out and the vessel collapses. The needle is often held best in the jaws of a haemostatic forceps (Fig. 104).

Advancing catheters

Whenever possible use a smooth ended catheter that does not tend to catch in irregularities along the inner wall of the duct or vessel. A fairly stiff, or even rigid, cannula must be used to pass between walls that have collapsed against each other, or are covered with sticky mucus. A soft and flexible catheter passes most easily along a channel that is distended with fluid. When circumstances allow it, smear lubricating substances on the catheter.

When the lumen is tortuous, straighten it whenever possible by stretching the duct. If the lumen cannot be straightened, use a catheter that almost fills the duct; a too thin catheter may turn upon itself. When advancing a flexible catheter along a tortuous channel,

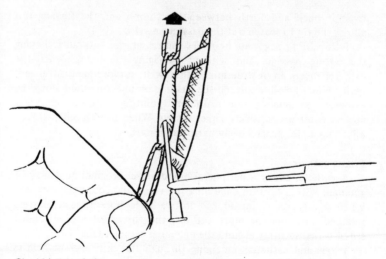

Fig. 104 Cannulating a very fine vessel with a needle mounted in a haemostatic forceps.

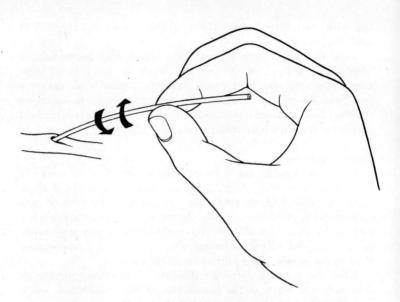

Fig. 105 Spin the catheter back and forth between the thumb and fingers, to allow it to search out the channel.

twist it back and forth between the thumb and the fingers; this allows the tip to search out the passageway (Fig. 105).

Take care to negotiate branches and tributaries without following the wrong passage, and without damaging the lining. When the catheter meets an obstruction, withdraw it, rotate it, and advance it again. When possible distend the channel by injecting fluid along the catheter. Remember that catheters pointing centrally in blood vessels enter progressively larger vessels. When introduced peripherally, they enter progressively narrower vessels.

Fixing catheters

A catheter filling a peripheral blood vessel or small duct may be retained with a ligature encircling the vessel and contained catheter. When a catheter is introduced into a wide bore tube it may be retained with one or more sutures; the thread of the outermost stitch is tied securely around the emerging catheter (Fig. 106).

Tubes and catheters emerging through the skin may be held in place with strips of adhesive plaster or tape. A stitch through the skin may transfix the tube but if leakage must be avoided the ends

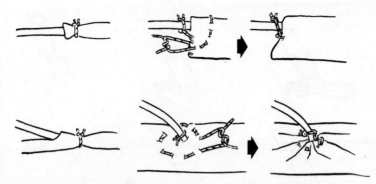

Fig. 106 Fixing catheters into small ducts on the left, and into large ducts on the right.

of thread are tied several times around the tube (Fig. 107). An elastic catheter can be fixed by cutting off a short length, stretching it over the main tube to form a tight collar, and stitching this to the skin.

Dilatation of ducts

Natural channels require dilatation as a rule only as the result of damage or disease with stricture formation. Occasionally normal channels are deliberately dilated for convenient passage of substances into them.

Dilators are rods of circular cross-section. They may be of rigid metal or semi-rigid gum-elastic and plastic. Dilators may be straight or curved. Rigid instruments are more damaging in clumsy hands but when skilfully used give a better 'feel', and the direction can be controlled. Malleable instruments are useful if the shape of the track is not known.

The tip of a dilator is rounded and of smaller diameter than the shank, the transition being gentle. Once the tip has entered a stricture, advancing the dilator gradually stretches it. An olivary-tipped dilator has an oval globular end, likened to an olive. As the olive slips through the stricture its onward passage becomes suddenly easier, giving an estimate of the length of stricture. The length can be confirmed by withdrawing the olive, noting when the grip of the stricture is suddenly relaxed. The freedom of the dilator when the tip has passed the stricture allows the 'feel' to be retained. The proximal segment has an expanding diameter which dilates the stricture.

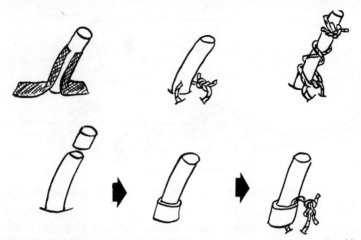

Fig. 107 On the top row are shown methods of fixing catheters to the skin using adhesive plaster or stitches. On the bottom row is shown a method (suggested by Miss Phyllis George) using a collar cut from the catheter, slipped over it, and stitched to the skin.

Start with the largest dilator that is likely to pass. When circumstances permit, apply a lubricant such as liquid paraffin or water-soluble jelly. If possible, straighten the passage by applying traction to one end.

Never use force to drive the tip of the dilator through the stricture. Try varying the direction of the tip until it engages. If this fails, then try successively smaller instruments. Misdirected force creates a false passage that will abort future attempts to dilate the stricture.

MULTIPLE STRICTURES require great sensitivity of touch to negotiate. The grip upon the instrument of the first stricture or a tight orifice, dulls the sense of 'feel' of the tip. Whenever possible dilate each stricture sufficiently to allow the instrument to lie freely when it reaches the next one.

FALSE PASSAGES. Ducts opening into the main channel, or holes created by previous rough dilatations may lead the tip of the dilator out of the main channel into a cul de sac. Withdraw the dilator, and advance it while keeping the tip pressed against the opposite wall of the duct. Occasionally one dilator can be left in the false passage to block its mouth while a second instrument passes along the main channel.

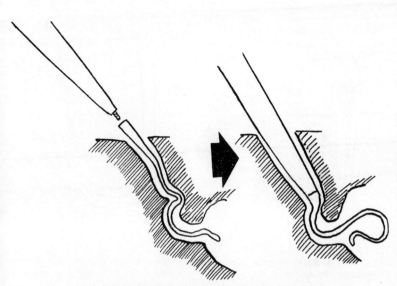

Fig. 108 Using a filiform leader as a pilot for the dilator.

FILIFORM LEADER. When a dilator cannot be passed, a fine flexible bougie may be induced to follow a tortuous path through a stricture. The dilator is then attached to the pilot bougie and acts as a leader for it (Fig. 108). The flexibility of the leader allows it to fold upon itself. Occasionally the end of a cotton or linen thread will be carried through a stricture by peristalsis or fluid flow. If the thread can be recovered at the other end of the stricture, it may also act as a leader (Fig. 109); thicker thread may be attached and drawn through, and subsequently this can be tied to the end of a dilator to draw it through the stricture.

TECHNIQUE OF DILATATION. When the first dilator has negotiated the stricture, take note of its pathway. Do not remove it until the next larger size is to hand. Draw the first dilator out and swiftly and smoothly replace it with the next size, repeating this until the desired amount of dilatation is achieved. The end of each bigger dilator is slightly smaller than the shank of the preceding one.

The direction of the end of a rigid dilator is controlled by movement of the handle end (Fig. 110). The direction of insertion is noted, confirmed during the withdrawal and repeated for the next dilator. By maintaining traction on the duct, the track can often be straightened.

99

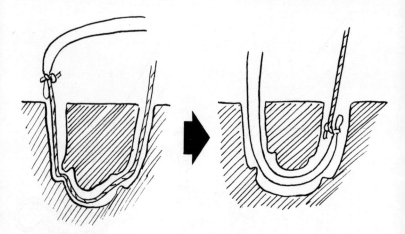

Fig. 109 A thread end has been induced to pass the stricture and acts as a leader for the dilator.

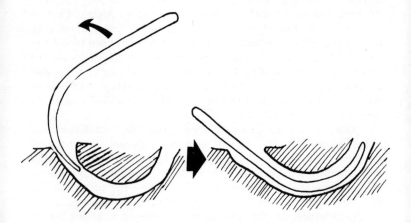

Fig. 110 Negotiating a curved channel with a rigid curved dilator. The handle of the dilator must be swung in an arc to direct the point along the curved path.

To confirm the negotiation of a stricture in a curved duct while using a rigid curved dilator that enters a wider channel, try rotating the dilator. It cannot rotate if the end still lies within the narrow duct, but it can do so if it has reached the wide channel beyond. This is used when dilating urethral strictures to confirm that the bladder has been reached.

EXTENT OF DILATATION. In many circumstances the channel is to be dilated but once. When an epithelial lined duct is dilated to overcome stricture formation, the stretching must be gentle and progressive. Repeated dilatations, gaining a little each time, are better than a single forcible stretching. The aim of gentle dilatation is to stretch the subepithelial fibrous tissue whilst leaving the lining intact. If the epithelium is split, as signalled by the presence of blood on the dilator as it is withdrawn, further scar tissue will be formed and undergo contraction resulting in even tighter stricture formation. Do not, therefore, attempt to attain the final duct calibre at a single dilatation in the presence of a severe stricture.

Never fail to record the sizes of dilators passed, with details of difficulties that may be helpful at subsequent dilatations.

Occlusion of ducts and vessels

OPEN END. The vessel or duct may need to be divided or have been divided accidentally.

Ligature. A blood vessel or small duct can be occluded by constricting the lumen with a ligature. Do not place the ligature too near the end, otherwise it may slip off (Fig. 73). A ligature is conveniently placed by first catching the end of the vessel with haemostatic forceps and applying the ligature below this, then removing the forceps. Large vessels should be doubly ligated for extra safety.

Transfixion ligature. To prevent a ligature from slipping off the end of an occluded vessel, first carry it through the vessel mounted on a needle, then encircle the vessel and tie the ligature (Fig. 74).

Metal clips. In certain situations small metal clips, carried in a special holder, are clamped across the ends of small vessels to occlude them.

Diathermization. If a high frequency alternating electric current is passed through the body tissues it generates heat. An electrode in contact with a wide area diffuses the heat but a small electrode concentrates the heat. Small blood vessels can be sealed by coagulating them with diathermy. Pick up the blood vessel with

101

forceps and touch this with the active electrode and switch on the current for just sufficient time to coagulate the vessel.

Twisting. Small vessels can be occluded by clamping them with haemostatic forceps, twisting them several turns and removing the forceps.

Purse-string suture. Large bore supple ducts such as bowel can be closed with a simple ligature or suture of the flattened end, followed by invagination within a purse-string suture applied around the bowel (Fig. 75).

Terminal suture. A rigid wide-bore tube cannot be constricted by a ligature, nor invaginated. It must be flattened while multiple sutures are placed along the edges to close it (Fig. 111).

IN CONTINUITY. If it is unnecessary or undesirable to divide a vessel or duct to occlude it, a ligature can be tied around it. Large and rigid channels cannot be so occluded but must be divided, with flattening and suture of the ends. Double ligatures, spaced apart, discourage recanalization, but this can be prevented with certainty only by dividing the duct between the ligatures, and separating the ends.

Control of leakage

Blood vessels and ducts can be temporarily occluded, sometimes without displaying them, by compressing them against a firm background with fingers. If a vessel has been displayed and mobilized, it may be compressed between finger and thumb.

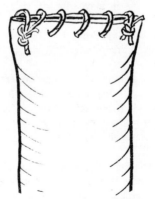

Fig. 111 Closing a wide bore tube with a row of sutures after flattening the end.

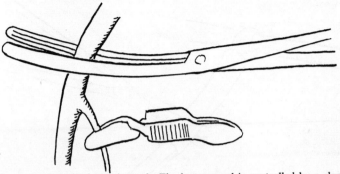

Fig. 112 Control of blood vessels. The larger vessel is controlled by a clamp which can be closed. The smaller vessel is controlled by a spring 'bulldog' clamp.

A pinching action can be reproduced by applying a clamp which will occlude the lumen without damaging the walls (Fig. 112). Vessels and ducts with supple walls can be controlled by encircling them with a thread or tape tied but not tightened with a half hitch. A thin-walled vessel may be occluded by pulling upon the thread and angulating the vessel. Alternatively the thread or tape ends can be led through a section of rubber tubing; the vessel is occluded by pulling upon the thread ends, and placing a clamp across the rubber tube (Fig. 113).

Disobliteration

The lumen of some ducts which have become obstructed can subsequently be opened up. When wide and supple ducts are occluded by disease affecting the wall, part of the wall can be excised, or a complete segment can be resected and the ends joined together. A narrow section of a supple wide bore duct can be widened by making a longitudinal incision through the stricture which is divided longitudinally; this incision is widely opened and then closed as a transverse suture line, producing a wider, but shorter segment (Fig. 114).

Narrow segments of smaller ducts, including blood vessels, must be excised with end to end union, or the interposition of a graft or tube of artificial material. If the duct is cut transversely the resulting circumferential suture line may form a narrowing. It is therefore wise to cut and suture such ducts obliquely (Fig. 115). Alternatively a patch may be inserted.

103

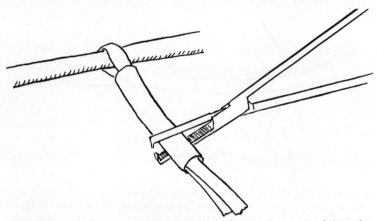

Fig. 113 Controlling a blood vessel. The tape encircles the vessel and the ends are passed through rubber tubing. If the tape ends are pulled tight and forceps are clamped across the tubing, the blood vessel will be occluded.

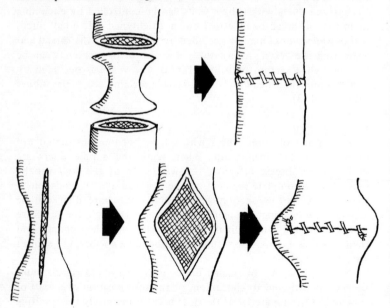

Fig. 114 Top. The stricture has been excised and the two ends are joined. Bottom. A longitudinal incision is opened out and stitched up as a transverse suture line.

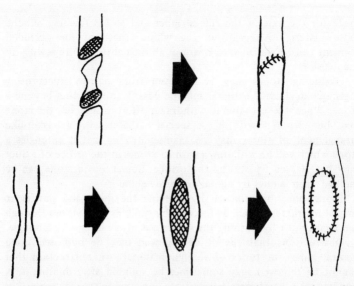

Fig. 115 Top: the stenosed segment is excised; the obliquely cut ends are then joined together. Bottom: the longitudinal incision through the strictured segment is opened out and a patch graft is inserted.

Intraluminal obstruction of a large duct by a foreign body, inspissated contents, stones, worms and flukes, can be relieved by incising the duct over the obstruction and removing the debris and closing the duct. Blood vessels occluded by clot or atheromatous plaques may be opened at a convenient point to allow the lumen to be cleared. An embolus or recently formed blood clot can sometimes be removed with a Fogarty catheter, which is a thin, flexible tube carrying an inflatable balloon near its tip. The catheter is inserted through a small incision in the vessel wall, is passed through the clot until it reaches unobstructed vessel lumen. The balloon is inflated with fluid to fill the lumen, and the catheter is withdrawn, acting as a piston to draw out the contents. The catheter may be repassed and used to flush the remaining debris clear, after which the incision is closed.

Atheromatous material can be cleared from a blood vessel only by removing the degenerated intimal lining. A ring of the correct size, mounted on a shaft, is inserted through an incision and can be pushed along the lumen of the vessel, separating the obstructing material so that it can be flushed out. A second incision may be

105

made for the exit of the ring stripper and to aid flushing out the loose material. Alternatively the whole length of the occluded segment can be slit open to clear out all the debris, before sewing up the incision.

Occluding stones may be removed from narrow ducts using ingenious devices. A catheter may be passed into the duct beyond a stone. When the catheter is withdrawn after an interval, the stone may be extruded with it. A special catheter with a basket-like arrangement of fibres may be manipulated so that it entangles a stone which will be withdrawn with it. Stones at the orifice of a duct may be released by slitting the orifice. Sometimes a stone can be 'milked' from a duct by digital pressure behind it.

Stones may be removed by opening the duct, and passing in special instruments such as forceps, by 'milking' the stones through the incision, or by pushing the stones out of the duct with a bougie.

Obstructions that cannot be removed may be bypassed using natural tubes, or tubes of foreign material. An obstruction that cannot be removed may sometimes be splinted after dilating it. A non-irritant tube of metal or plastic is impacted in the stricture.

Repair

Large ducts are repaired using stitches suited to their size. Bowel is usually sewn with chromicized catgut swaged into eyeless needles; the stitches are taken through all layers of the bowel, and it is orthodox practice to invert the bowel wall, bringing into apposition the serous coats, reinforcing the inversion with a second layer of stitches that picks up the seromuscular layers.

Blood vessels are repaired using a single layer of fine black silk sutures swaged onto small eyeless needles. To keep the lining in contact with blood as smooth as possible the endothelial surfaces are apposed by everting the vessel wall. Arterial and vein grafts or patches may be inserted, or plastic tubes used to bridge gaps in large blood vessels.

Certain ducts, such as bile ducts that may have lost their inner lining, can be repaired over tubes that will either be left in place as splints to prevent scarring and consequent stenosis at the anasto-mosis or will later be removed.

Individual nerve sheaths cannot be united but nerves are repaired by placing fine stitches of non-reactive material through the perineural connective tissue sheath to unite cut nerves, after ensuring that the cut ends are in correct alignment.

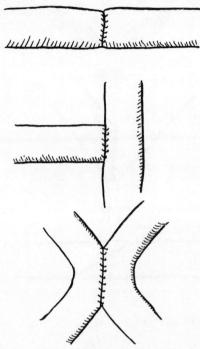

Fig. 116 At top, an end to end anastomosis. At centre, an end to side anastomosis. At bottom, a side to side anastomosis.

Anastomosis

Ducts and vessels may be joined to leave a passage for the transmission of contents, either to repair them after damage and resection of disease, or in order to rechannel the contents.

Large ducts such as bowel may be joined end to end, end to side, or side to side (Fig. 116). A side to side anastomosis can be made of unlimited size. The bowel edges are inverted with an all-coats stitch, reinforced with a second seromuscular stitch. This inversion temporarily narrows the lumen although final remodelling leaves minimal stenosis. To avoid temporary obstruction of narrow ducts, the anastomosis should be made larger than the lumen of the bowel. When the end of a duct is used, it should be cut obliquely (Fig. 117). Bowel is left longer at the mesenteric border, where the blood vessels enter, to protect against ischaemia.

Smaller ducts and blood vessels are usually joined in a single

107

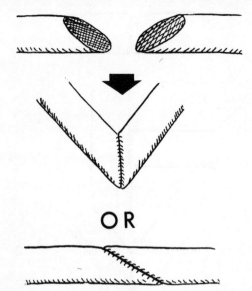

Fig. 117 Small ducts are cut obliquely so that the anastomosis does not encircle the bowel and obstruct it.

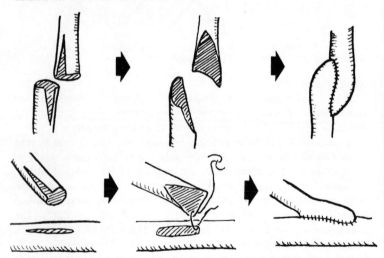

Fig. 118 Top: two small ducts or vessels are united after slitting the ends and opening them out to create a wide anastomosis. Bottom: a small duct or vessel has been slit before joining it into the side of a large duct or vessel.

layer. Blood vessel edges are everted to ensure an intact endothelial lining is in contact with the blood. In order to make the anastomosis as large as possible, small vessels are united by joining the ends after making a longitudinal slit in the wall and opening out the vessel (Fig. 118).

When a small duct is to be joined to a larger duct, part of the end of the large duct may be closed until the remaining lumen matches that of the smaller duct. Alternatively the end of the large duct is completely closed and the small duct is joined to a small side hole in the large duct (Fig. 119). Very small ducts may be joined by first cannulating them with a plastic catheter which is tied in. The end of the catheter is inserted into the recipient duct or organ, carrying the end of the duct. One end of the ligature is threaded onto a needle which is taken into the hole receiving the duct and out again, to be

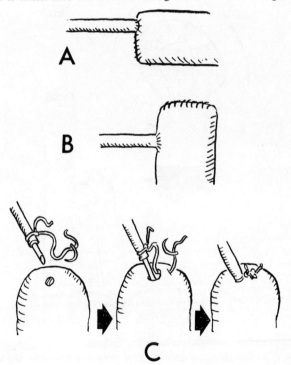

Fig. 119 Joining small ducts into large vessels. A, End to end. B, End to side. C, Using a plastic cannula to aid the union of a small duct to a large vessel.

tied to the other end of the ligature. The join may be reinforced by inserting a purse string suture to invaginate the hole in the recipient organ or duct.

Nerves are joined end to end, stitching the perineurium only.

Transplantation

When bowel or other large ducts with a rich blood supply are to be used in a different situation, they must retain a blood supply or they will die. It is often possible to extend a loop of bowel while preserving its blood supply by utilizing the arching blood vessels that run in the mesentery, so that blood vessels supply it from one end while the other end is stretched out (Fig. 120). If the bowel is to be

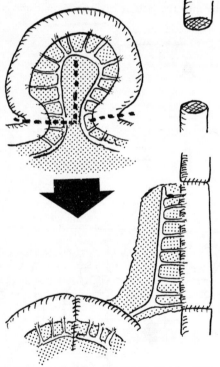

Fig. 120 Transplanting bowel while retaining its blood supply. At the top the dotted line shows the line of section. The loop is opened out and anastomosed in the lower diagram.

used at a distance or be transplanted to another recipient then the major blood vessels must be successfully united to vessels at the recipient site, and all minor cut vessels are closed.

Arteries and veins are nourished from blood flowing through them, so that they may be freely transplanted. Veins may be used to replace sections of arteries. If valved veins are used, they are reversed so that the valves do not impede blood flow. Stenosed arteries can therefore be replaced or bypassed using arterial grafts, vein grafts, or artificial tubes. The smallness of arteries that can be united is not limited by technical difficulties, but when small vessels are joined, the relatively slow rate of blood flow and the small anastomosis, make thrombosis and obstruction very likely.

Small ducts such as the ureter are supplied with blood vessels at intervals. They should not be too freely mobilized when being diverted, in case the blood supply is prejudiced.

Segments of peripheral nerves may be freely transplanted. It is not the nerve fibres but the nerve sheaths that are needed in the new site to form conduits for the regenerating proximal fibres trying to rejoin their end organs.

Sinus and fistulous tracks may be joined into normal ducts in order to provide a drainage channel for them.

Sphincters

Control of fluid flow through ducts is often achieved in otherwise passive conduits such as blood vessels by constriction along the length of the vessel. In other tubes, such as the bowel, localized areas of principally circular muscle control the rate and direction of flow, called sphincters. These may be anatomically obvious or deduced from functional studies.

Take care to anticipate sphincters and their nerve and blood supplies when dissecting, since inadvertent damage may be irrevocable. However, for functional reasons, direct operations may be performed on sphincters.

DILATATION. A sphincter may be dilated using graduated instruments in the same manner as a strictured duct is dilated. An empty hollow bag is sometimes placed within the sphincter and distended with air or water to stretch it. If the intention is to restore the lumen to normal, take care not to overstretch and paralyse the sphincter.

Sometimes the sphincter is deliberately overstretched to paralyse it temporarily or permanently. Even in these circumstances do not

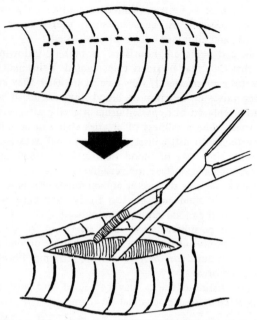

Fig. 121 Myotomy. The sphincter is divided (top) along the dotted line. The edges are split apart (bottom) to ensure that all the circular muscle is divided.

act roughly; if the duct lining is torn, fibrous healing and contracture may subsequently narrow the lumen through the sphincter.

MYOTOMY. Clearly defined circular muscle forming a sphincter may be divided by a longitudinal incision along the duct without necessarily opening the lumen of the duct (Fig. 121). This permanently destroys the sphincteric action.

Hold the portion of duct steady with fingers, or grasp it using encircling tissue forceps, trying to place the circular fibres on the superior aspect under tension by angulating the duct up towards you. Cut carefully using a scalpel allowing the tension in the deeper parts of the cut to separate the edges. As soon as the muscle is transected and the lining bulges into the wound, stop cutting. Make sure that no fibres have been missed, especially at the limits of the transphincteric incision. Gently lift intact fibres using a hook or fine non-toothed forceps and cut through them. If the muscle ring is sufficiently thick, any few remaining fibres can be gently broken by picking up each side of the cut edge with fingers, using gauze swabs to improve the grip, and separating the edges. Alternatively, round-nosed artery forceps can be used to lever the edges apart. Ensure that the lining is intact so that no leakage occurs. In relatively empty parts of the gut it may still be possible to trap a little air into the sphincteric segment and compress it, to check that none leaks out. If there is a leak, close it now, covering the repair with another layer of tissue if possible—in the case of bowel, pull an edge of omentum over the area and stitch it in place.

SPHINCTEROTOMY. The whole thickness of the sphincter, together with the vessel or duct lining, can be divided in some circumstances, for instance when the sphincter controls the termination of a spouted duct (Fig. 122). Sometimes it is possible to insinuate one blade of scissors into the lumen and then cut through. Alternatively, pass a grooved probe into the duct and cut down into

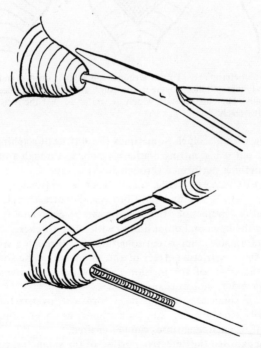

Fig. 122 Sphincterotomy. Top: one blade of the scissors is passed up the duct to cut the sphincter. Bottom: a grooved probe passed up the duct to guide the tip of a scalpel cutting through the sphincter.

113

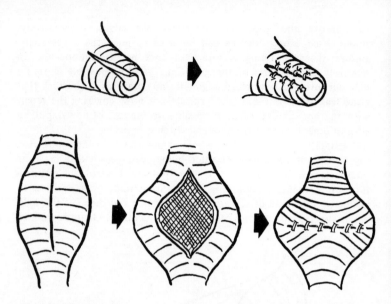

Fig. 123 Sphincteroplasty. Top: a terminal sphincter is divided and the inner and outer linings stitched together. Bottom: a sphincter has been divided longitudinally. The cut edges are widely separated so that the incision can be sutured transversely.

the groove with a scalpel. Sometimes the slitting of a sphincter may be carried out using cutting diathermy applied through a fine point; this is sometimes performed through an endoscope.

SPHINCTEROPLASTY. (Fig. 123). When a terminal sphincter is divided and left, it may undergo fibrosis and contraction. In the case of a spoutlike projection, the fibrosis can be considerably reduced by uniting the inner and outer linings with a few stitches.

If a deformable duct is cut longitudinally through a sphincteric segment, the constricting effect of the sphincter can be annulled by opening the edges of the incision and sewing it transversely. This results in a wider, shorter channel.

REPAIR. A sphincter that has been torn, cut, overstretched, or is congenitally incomplete, can sometimes be made functionally effective if its encircling fibres can be repaired.

Having exposed the defective portion of the sphincter, cut cleanly through it on each side of the defect, taking care to tag each of the exposed structures with marker stitches or fine tissue forceps. Plan to cut a 'V' out of a terminal sphincter, and an ellipse out of a sphincter in continuity with the duct (Fig. 124).

Repair the sphincter from within outwards, starting with the lining, then proceed to the individual muscle bundles, ensuring that they are correctly aligned with each other.

Whenever possible, arrange to relax and rest the sphincter during the period of healing.

REVERSAL. Some sphincters are unidirectional in action like valves, allowing flow only one way along the duct. The duct may be transected at each end of the sphincter, retaining the blood and nerve supply to the sphincteric section. If the sphincter is now reversed and restored in continuity with the duct, its action upon the duct contents will be reversed (Fig. 125).

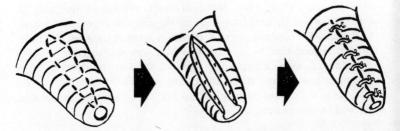

Fig. 124 Repair of sphincter. Stretched portion excised (dotted line) and resulting fresh sphincter muscle edges sutured together to restore the sphincteric action.

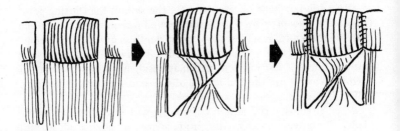

Fig. 125 Sphincter reversal. The sphincteric segment is freed but retains its nerve and blood supply. It is reversed and sutured into place, thus reversing its action.

115

Chapter 5

HANDLING SKIN

Elastic tissue makes skin resilient and conform to underlying structures. The elasticity disappears in old age and disease. Tension is not equal in all directions but tends to run parallel to the creases seen at joints (Fig. 126). Incisions made parallel to the lines of tension show little tendency to gape, the edges re-appose easily, and heal well with minimal scarring. Incisions made at right angles to the lines of tension tend to gape and may heal with scarring.

Inflamed skin appears red, feels hot, and is swollen from accumulation of interstitial fluid. The surface is tethered at hair follicles and the orifices of sweat glands, giving a pitted appearance likened to orange peel.

Incision

Decide the correct line, taking into consideration the structure to be displayed, the intervening tissues, the tension lines of the skin, and the cosmetic importance of the scar. If the incision is complicated, mark it out using contrasting dye.

Using the left hand, stretch and fix the skin at the starting point (Fig. 127). Except when a short stab wound is required, cut with the belly of the knife, reaching the correct depth as quickly as possible. The scalpel cuts best when the sharp edge is drawn across the tissues; static pressure is less efficient and may result in an uneven depth of cutting. Always use the full length of the skin incision, so avoiding half-incised ends.

When circumstances permit, cut boldly, with a single sweep of the blade. Tentative scratchy cuts produce ragged, oozing edges with small half-detached pieces that will undergo necrosis and delay healing (Fig. 128). Scissors are occasionally preferable to a scalpel for cutting flaps of skin, provided the blades are rigid and remain in contact; if they separate the skin is crushed.

116

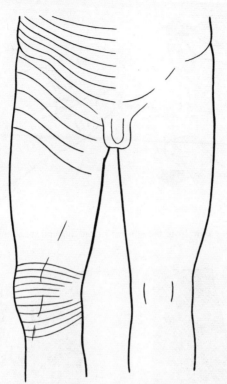

Fig. 126 Tension lines tend to run parallel to the creases seen at joints.

Control initial oozing from the cut surfaces by pressing with your finger tips along one edge, while your assistant presses on the opposite edge (Fig. 129). Use folded gauze swabs if necessary. Severe oozing can be diminished by applying artery forceps at intervals of about a centimetre, to the deep part of the cut skin edges. Lay the forceps handles on the intact surface to evert the skin edges (Fig. 130). The oozing will moderate very quickly. Individual vessels may be picked up with fine artery forceps, twisted, and released. If possible avoid ligatures since they impair wound healing. Diathermy current should be used sparingly, since skin burns heal slowly. It is permissible to coagulate deep dermal vessels provided they are picked up with fine forceps, and provided the current is switched to 'cutting' and is applied at the lowest possible intensity for the shortest possible time.

117

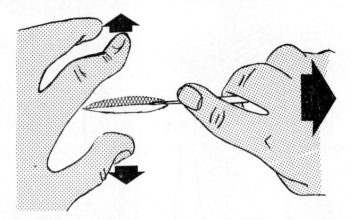

Fig. 127 Incising skin. Note the left hand steadying and spreading the skin.

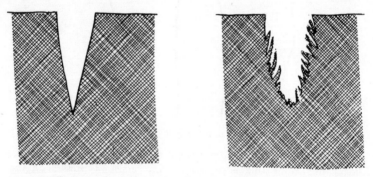

Fig. 128 Diagrammatic views of incisions. On the left the incision is cleanly made with one stroke. On the right multiple cuts have produced ragged edges.

Closure

A simple incision is closed by re-apposing the edges of skin that were separated. Healing cannot take place between the superficial dead keratinized layers, so inversion of the edges must be prevented. It is the deep germinal layers that must be accurately apposed, so the skin should be very slightly everted (Fig. 131). Skin is usually closed using non-absorbable thread in a contrasting colour to skin, mounted on straight or curved cutting-edged needles. Simple stitches may be used provided the edges are slightly everted as the needle penetrates

118

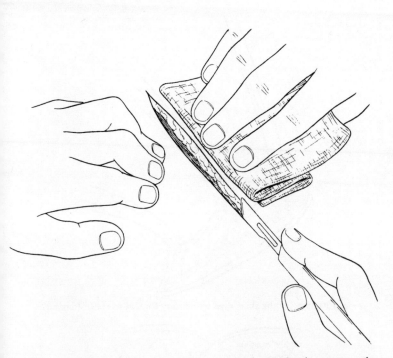

Fig. 129 The operator's left hand and the assistant's right hand press upon the skin edges to reduce oozing after incising the skin.

them. The edges can be everted using forceps or skin hooks, though simple pressure with closed forceps suffices (Fig. 132). If the edges have a marked tendency to invert, use a horizontal or vertical mattress stitch (Fig. 133). Tie the stitches just tight enough to unite the edges. The more evenly-tensioned sutures that are inserted, the less the traction on each stitch. For the best cosmetic result, insert stitches at intervals of 3–4 mm, placed a similar distance from the skin edges.

Metal clips taken from a gallery fitted to toothed forceps and inserted using special holding forceps, have an everting action on the skin. Apply them from right to left, holding the carrier in the left hand (Fig. 134). Grip the apposed edges and draw them to the right with the right hand forceps. Grip the edges together with the left hand forceps, now drawing the wound to the left. With the right hand forceps lift a clip from the carrier, apply it across the wound

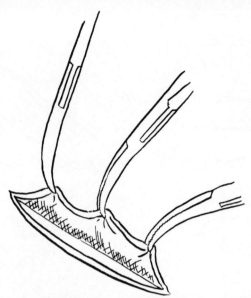

Fig. 130 Everting the skin edges with artery forceps to control oozing.

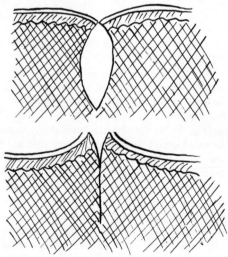

Fig. 131 The upper diagram shows inverted skin edges. The dead keratinized layers are in contact. The lower diagram shows everted skin edges. The live germinal layers are in contact and the edges will rapidly fuse.

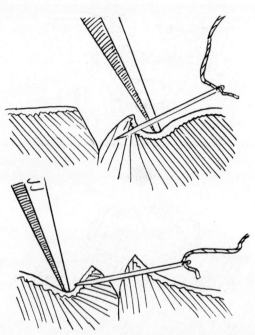

Fig. 132 Everting the skin edges while stitching them. Closed dissecting forceps pressed upon the skin everts the edge and steadies it against the thrust of the needle.

just to the right of the left hand forceps. Compress the clip, retaining a grip upon it, so that it can be drawn firmly to the right to tauten the wound. Release the left hand forceps and apply them just to the left of the chosen site of the next clip. Draw the wound to the left, releasing the grip of the right hand forceps, which apply the next clip. Continue in this manner to the end of the wound.

When it is important to prevent stitch or clip holes in the skin, use a subcuticular stitch, provided the wound is straight. After piercing the skin from one end with a needled thread, take bites of the deep cuticular edges from within the wound, making sure that the thread crosses the wound at right angles to the edges (Fig. 135). When the last stitch has been inserted, pierce the skin so that the thread emerges clear of the wound. If the two ends are gently pulled apart, the wound edges are apposed. The thread can subsequently be removed by pulling the ends alternately until the thread is freed and can be drawn out.

121

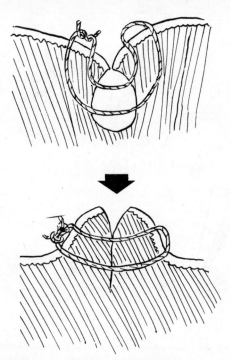

Fig. 133 The everting effect of correctly inserted mattress stitches.

As an alternative to stitches, adhesive strips may be applied across the wound to appose the edges (Fig. 135). Unless they adhere right up to the edges of the skin, they have an inverting effect, so do not use them to close oozing wounds, and ensure that the skin is absolutely dry before applying them.

Whenever possible avoid closing skin under excessive tension. If skin has been lost, spread the tension by undercutting the edges (Fig. 136). If the base is relatively avascular, the undercut skin must retain its subcutaneous blood supply. If the base is vascular, the skin may be better apposed if fatty avascular subcutaneous tissue is removed. To dissect off the subcutaneous tissue, evert the skin at first with dissecting forceps and later with fingers (Fig. 137), if necessary using gauze swabs to improve the grip. Cut evenly with a sharp scalpel just below the dermis, exposing it as a white, opaque layer, free of fat. To avoid cutting 'buttonholes' in the skin, constantly test the remaining thickness.

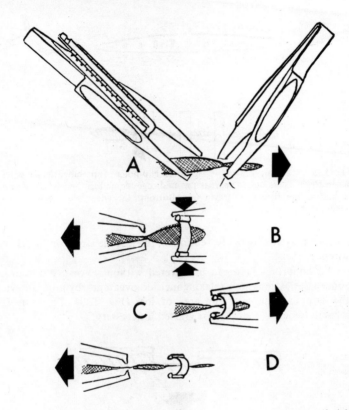

Fig. 134 Inserting Michel clips. A, Right hand forceps grasp apposed right hand skin edges and draws them to the right while left hand forceps grip skin. B, left hand forceps draw apposed skin edges to left. Right hand forceps remove a clip from the gallery on left hand forceps, and apply it across the skin edges. C, Right hand forceps compress clip, retaining their grip to draw the clip to the right. D, Left hand forceps take a fresh grip and draw skin to the left. Right hand forceps relax their grip ready to apply the next clip.

When forced by circumstances to close skin under greater than normal tension, or when the length of the edges to be apposed are incongruous, partially appose the edges with guide stitches that will later be removed. Place the first of these between the middles of the apposing edges, then place others halving the intervening spaces (Fig. 138). Insert the definitive stitches and then remove the guide stitches, which will by this time have become slack. The more

123

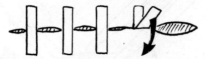

Fig. 135 Skin closure avoiding stitch or clip holes. Top: subcuticular stitch. When the ends are pulled apart the wound edges come together. When one end is pulled, the thread is drawn out. Bottom: the edges are apposed using adherent strips of tape.

stitches that are correctly tensioned, the less the strain on individual stitches.

An important area can be covered without excessive tension in some cases by making a relaxing incision over a nearby area, allowing the skin to slide over the area of loss (Fig. 139). This leaves a secondary defect that may be grafted if necessary.

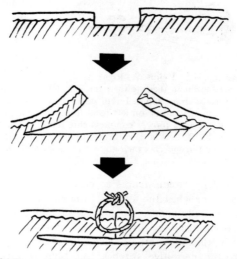

Fig. 136 To avoid stitching skin under tension, undercut the edges.

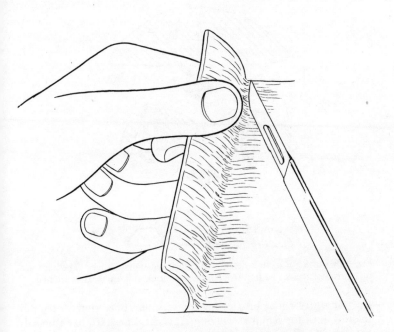

Fig. 137 Undercutting skin after everting the edge.

Grafts

These can be cut from one area of skin and used to cover defects elsewhere.

A split skin, or Thiersch graft includes the superficial layers of the skin, but with some germinal cells. It will survive where the blood supply of the recipient site is relatively poor. Stretch the donor area to make it flat and as rigid as possible. Hold a board in the left hand, with the edge pressed against the skin, drawing it towards you before the approach of the knife. If necessary get an assistant to draw the skin in the opposite direction (Fig. 140). Hold the previously lubricated graft knife flat and cut the skin with a sawing motion, concentrating on an even, short, stroke. Do not press too hard and do not angle the knife against the skin, or it will cut right through.

125

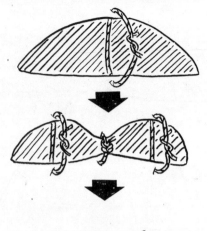

Fig. 138 Closing a gaping defect with disproportionate edges. The gaps are successively halved. The first stitches become slack as more stitches are tied.

Do not worry about progressing too fast, and once started, try not to stop until the required size of graft is cut. The graft, like thin soft paper, will accumulate in folds on the blade of the knife. The base will appear initially opaquely white, soon to develop petechial

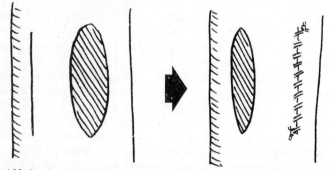

Fig. 139 On the left a defect cannot be closed without excessive tension. An incision has been made parallel to it. On the right the skin has been slid over to cover the defect, opening a defect at the site of the relaxing incision which may be closed by undermining the edge or by applying a skin graft.

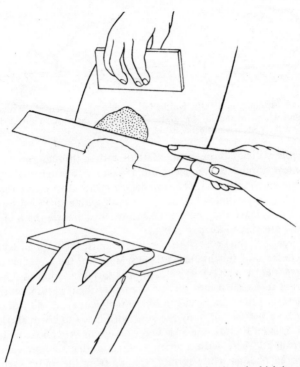

Fig. 140 Cutting a split skin graft. The left hand holds a board which is pressed on the skin and draws it taut before the knife. The graft knife is held in the right hand. The skin graft is cut using a back and forth motion of the knife. The assistant steadies and tautens the skin using a second board, at the top of the drawing.

haemorrhages if the depth of cut is correct. If the cut is too shallow, the graft will be incomplete and the knife will cut out. If the graft is too thick, subcutaneous fat will be seen. When sufficient area has been cut, raise the knife horizontally to produce a vertical curtain of graft attached to the skin, and detach it with scissors.

Make sure you distinguish the outer keratinized surface of the graft which is dull, from the inner, shiny base. The base must be laid in contact with the recipient area. Lift the graft into place, spreading it and sliding it into position with the closed tips of fine, non-toothed dissecting forceps. Trim off the overlapping edges of the graft using scissors. If you intend to stitch the graft in place,

127

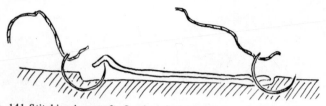

Fig. 141 Stitching in a graft. On the left the needle has pierced the intact skin first and is now dislodging the graft. On the right the stitch pierced the graft first and the graft has not been displaced.

insert the stitches through the graft first, then through the surviving skin edges around the recipient site. If you try to stitch the opposite way, the emerging needle tends to detach rather than pierce the graft (Fig. 141). If you intend to cover the graft with a shaped dressing to compress it, leave the ends of the sutures long and tie them together over the dressing to keep it in place.

A free full thickness graft, or Wolfe graft, includes all layers of the skin freed of subcutaneous tissues. Mark out the area that will be required before cutting it, since it will shrink as soon as it is free, requiring to be sewn into its new site under slight natural tension. A template of gauze can be cut to fit the recipient area, and laid on the donor area before outlining the skin with ink. Cut through the full depth of skin. Elevate one edge with forceps or skin hooks and cut it free from the base with a sharp scalpel, aiming to remove all fat, leaving an opaque white surface. Oozing from the under surface of the graft will quickly stop, but the donor site will ooze freely, requiring haemostasis.

Transfer the graft to the recipient site, which must have a suitable clean, vascular base. Sew in the corners first, to slightly stretch the graft, then progressively halve the unsewn areas. The donor site can sometimes be closed after undermining the edges, or by using a split skin graft.

If the recipient base for a full thickness graft is insufficiently vascular, and if the donor area can be brought close to it, a full thickness graft can be transferred, leaving one edge still attached as a pedicle through which the graft receives a blood supply until it becomes established in the new site, after which the attachment is divided.

Mark out the area to be elevated, including the extra portion of skin that will form the bridge between donor and recipient sites (Fig. 142). Cut through skin and subcutaneous tissue to the deep fascia,

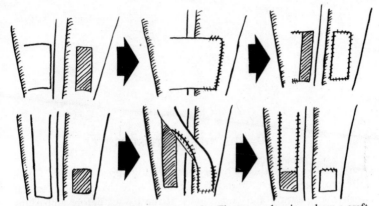

Fig. 142 Pedicled full thickness skin grafts. The upper drawings show a graft raised on the left, extended to cover a raw area in the centre, and divided from the established graft on the right. The uncovered donor area may be grafted with split skin. The lower drawings show the use of tubed pedicles. On the left a long graft is raised. In the centre the flap is swung to cover the defect. The bridge is converted into a tube, and the donor area may be temporarily closed. On the right the bridge is separated from the established graft, opened out, and replaced in its original bed.

and elevate the skin and subcutaneous tissue taking care not to carry the dissection into a more superficial plane as the flap is elevated. Bleeding occurs from the donor site and from the under surface of the graft. Catch vessels with fine artery forceps, and twist them, ligate them, or momentarily apply cutting diathermy current of low intensity.

Transfer the graft to the recipient site and sew it into position in the same manner as a free graft would be fixed, except that the side crossed by the bridging skin does not have an edge to sew into place.

After the graft has become established in its new site, a second operation will be performed to cut through the bridge, sew into place the resulting graft edge, and replace the bridge skin into place. The defect left by the graft is sutured after undermining the skin edges, or a split skin graft is applied.

In specially selected cases a pedicled graft, planned to retain a good vascular supply, can be swung to a distant donor site. The long bridge joining recipient and donor sites is temporarily formed into a tube with keratinized skin forming the outer layer. When the graft is established and detached, the tube is split along the suture line and replaced into its original bed.

Chapter 6

HANDLING SOFT TISSUES

Each of the body tissues has a characteristic appearance and feel at different ages, in health and disease. Make sure that you are familiar with the anatomy and consistency of the tissues before embarking on operations. The less they are damaged the quicker will they heal.

Some operators appear to charm tissues into obeying them; it is not magic, but thoughtful familiarity.

Connective tissue

This varies from flimsy areolar tissue to tough ligaments, tendons, and aponeuroses, depending upon the amount and disposition of collagenous and elastic fibres, and the presence or absence of fat. The vascularity also varies but the nutritional requirement of stable connective tissue is minimal; however, blood vessels may cross connective tissue spaces bound for other tissues and organs.

Flimsy connective tissue may be cut with scalpel or scissors. It can be repaired using fine, slightly chromicized catgut mounted on small round-bodied needles. Tough connective tissue is cut with a scalpel or heavy scissors. It is sutured using strong chromicized catgut or non-absorbable thread, mounted on stout cutting or trocar-pointed needles. If the fibres run predominantly in one direction, stitches must be inserted with care. When the connective tissue is cut across the fibres, join it with mattress sutures (Fig. 88). When the cut is parallel to the fibres, place the stitch-holes at varying distances from the edges to prevent a strip from being detached (Fig. 89).

Connective tissues heal slowly and the repair should be protected from strain when this is possible, until union is strong.

Skeletal muscle

This is remarkably fragile when relaxed. Because of the great metabolic requirements during muscular activity, the blood supply is generous. If the motor nerve supply is damaged the muscle will be paralysed. Muscle fibres are arranged parallel to each other in the direction of contraction, and they may be separated with minimal permanent damage; they can be re-apposed using chromicized catgut stitches mounted on round-bodied needles, tied loosely to avoid constricting the muscle fibres.

Muscles that have been cut across the fibres contract, separating the edges. If stitches are inserted they have a tendency to cut out between the fibres, so mattress stitches should be used. To minimize tension until the repair is sound, relax the muscle by immobilizing the part in a position that most nearly apposes the origin and insertion of the muscle. Healing will be by connective tissue, not by regeneration of the muscle fibres, so that if a single muscle belly is transected and repaired, a double-bellied muscle will result.

Tendons

These are composed of aligned collagen fibres, transmitting the pull of muscles. They may be split and will then heal without loss of strength but if they are transected the ends attached to the muscle retract. If the tendon is repaired the join is weak and stitches tend to cut out. Special criss-cross stitches of stainless steel are used (Fig. 90). Whenever possible the area of union is made as large as possible by cutting the ends obliquely or stepwise. During healing tension is kept to a minimum by immobilizing the part with the origin of the muscle and insertion of the tendon as close to each other as possible. The defect is repaired with collagen, and if it is strained it may stretch, with consequent limitation of muscle action.

Where a close-fitting tendon runs through a synovial sheath the irregularity resulting from a tendon repair may produce jerky movement. This can sometimes be minimized by arranging to remove the sutures when repair is complete.

The insertion of a tendon may be detached and reimplanted elsewhere, converting the pull of the muscle to a fresh action. Two or more tendons may be united, to give the attached muscle a double action. Important tendons may be repaired using grafts taken from less important tendons.

Cartilage

This may be cut with a scalpel, and stitched after drilling stitch holes. It usually heals by deposition of fibrocartilage. Cartilage may be transplanted from one part of the body to another.

131

Organs

Each organ has individual characteristics of appearance, consistency, vascularity, and ability to stand up to surgical manipulation. The brain is extremely delicate, but most other organs are remarkably tough and resistant to damage.

Some organs gain support from their fibrous capsules, such as liver, kidneys and spleen. The gut and lungs are mainly enclosed within the peritoneal and pleural membranes which have the property of rapidly sealing any defects. Glands such as the thyroid, pancreas and adrenals have minimal investing connective tissue capsules.

The viscera vary in their physical characteristics at different ages and in different subjects. Disease sometimes produces areas of softening or sclerosis in previously homogeneous organs. Inflammation, or overactivity may produce increased vascularity.

Before operating in the region of a viscus ensure that you are prepared by studying its blood supply and the anatomy of any ducts that are related to it. Never assume that it can be casually displaced, distorted, or incised.

LIVER is honeycombed with blood vessels and bile ducts, making it ooze blood and bile when cut or damaged. Stitches of chromicized catgut inserted on large, curved eyeless needles, must be placed well away from the edges and be tied just tightly enough to appose the edges, or they will cut out (Fig. 143). When making deliberate cuts

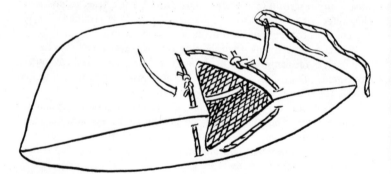

Fig. 143 Before sewing the liver edges together, using a large curved needle, preliminary constricting stitches have been inserted near the cut edges; these stop oozing and prevent the main stitches from cutting out.

into the liver the diathermy current may be used to reduce oozing, except when a specimen is needed for histology, which would be destroyed by heat. Alternatively the liver tissue may be bluntly dissected to display large vessels which are then clamped and divided.

SPLEEN notoriously continues to ooze whenever the capsule has been damaged. It is not repaired but is removed after ligating the splenic artery and vein.

KIDNEY has a generous blood supply. The capsule is tough and takes stitches well, so that a damaged kidney can be repaired provided the blood supply and urine drainage channel are intact.

PANCREAS is fragile, and when damaged releases digestive enzymes that destroy itself and surrounding tissues. Repair is difficult to achieve. The body and tail can be removed, closing the neck, and leaving the head intact. Cut the neck in a 'V' (Fig. 144), shorter in the central area, leaving the superficial parts longer. Sew them together like the parts of a fishtail to seal the gland against leakage.

UTERUS is a muscular organ, richly supplied with blood but especially so just before monthly periods and during pregnancy. The organ is tough and takes stitches well if it is cut and repaired.

OVARY AND TESTIS are well supplied with blood vessels and have strong fibrous capsules.

BLADDER is a hollow muscular organ that can be cut and stitched with catgut sutures.

LUNG is elastic and vascular, enclosed in the serous pleural membrane. It remains expanded by being enclosed within the negative-pressure potential space of the pleural cavity. If the lung is damaged air leaks into the cavity, allowing the lung to collapse. The lung is lobulated and segmented so that a portion can be excised, or the whole lung can be removed. The semirigid cartilagenous bronchi are closed by flattening them and inserting sutures of non-absorbent material, to keep the edges apposed (Fig. 111).

HEART is composed of tough, specialized muscle with intrinsic contractility. Techniques are available to stop the heart while

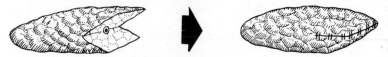

Fig. 144 On the left the pancreas has been cut like a fish tail. The duct is seen transected. After suturing the edges, the gland is sealed.

133

carrying out difficult intracardiac procedures and restart it subsequently—the pump action of the heart being taken over temporarily by a substitute pump. The heart muscle can be cut and sutured and will heal even though it is intermittently contracting throughout the period of healing.

BRAIN and spinal cord are almost fluid, behaving somewhat like a blancmange. If they are damaged, healing is by the deposition of connective glial tissue; the unmyelinated nerve fibres cannot reconnect. Nerve tracts can be divided within the brain and in the cord by direct approach, or occasionally by stereotactic surgery, with external control of the fibres to be divided. The brain is richly supplied with blood vessels; if they bleed the emerging blood causes local damage in addition to occupying the limited intracranial space, raising the pressure and causing further brain damage, often at a distance from the site of the bleed.

Chapter 7

HANDLING BONE

The bony skeleton demands different handling techniques from soft tissues. Bone is remarkably strong for its weight; by dynamic remoulding it adapts to the forces imposed upon it throughout life. During surgical operations it is often exposed to exceptional forces from unusual directions.

The techniques used for operating upon bone have almost without exception been adapted from carpentry, masonry, or engineering. Keep constantly in mind that smooth-grained wood, stone and metal for working, tend to be homogeneous, but bone is not. On the other hand, live bone has the capacity for self-healing.

Exposure

Plan the approach to produce the minimum damage. Whenever possible separate structures rather than divide them, remembering that overlying muscles must retain intact nerve and blood supplies if they are to function subsequently. Do not unnecessarily destroy or strip off the periosteum, since the deep layer is rich in osteoblasts; also the nutrient blood vessels reach the bone through the periosteum, and will be torn during stripping.

Steadying

Working with bone using sharp tools demands adequate steadiness, otherwise the bone will be damaged and the tools may slip and irrevocably destroy surrounding soft tissues. Make use of your assistant to hold limbs, retractors, levers, forceps, and gauze swabs, to fix the bone and protect other structures (Fig. 145).

Cutting

SAW. Decide the line of the cut. Ensure that the soft tissues are protected and will remain so throughout the manoeuvre. Remember

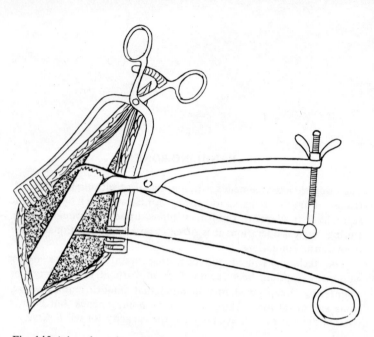

Fig. 145 A long bone is exposed using a self-retaining retractor to hold back the overlying tissues. It is steadied using bone-holding forceps, and lifted using a bone lever.

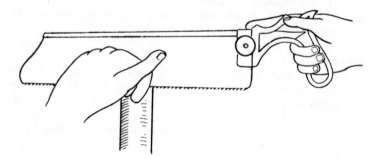

Fig. 146 To start cutting with a saw, steady the blade with the left thumb.

that a saw should be used to make straight cuts only; do not try to angle the blade during the procedure, but if necessary start a fresh cut. Remember that sawing removes bone—not just the thickness of the blade, but the width of the 'set' of the teeth.

Start the cut by gently drawing the saw towards you over the starting point, using the left thumb in contact with the blade well above the teeth, to steady it (Fig. 146).

A sharp saw cuts best if it is given an even, rhythmic, oscillating motion in the correct line, using the longest possible stroke, avoiding pressure that will cause the teeth to jam. When completing the cut, reduce the pressure to a minimum so that you do not cut too far. When completely sectioning bone make sure there is no strain across the diminishing isthmus of bone joining the two parts, or it will crack irregularly across. If possible make a small counter-cut through the opposite cortex of the bone, so that the break occurs away from the edge, avoiding a sharp projecting splinter.

When using powered tools, such as a circular saw, be doubly careful because the cut may rapidly over-run the desired course. Remember also that the part of the blade that is cutting into bone is not the only part that can do damage.

CHISEL (Fig. 147). A chisel is bevelled on one side and is principally used for shaping bone. If a cut is angled into the bony structure with

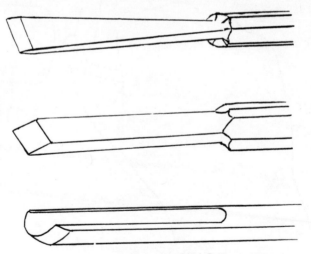

Fig. 147 Top, osteotome. Centre, chisel, Bottom, gouge.

the bevel uppermost, the cut becomes progressively deeper whereas it tends to cut out when the straight edge is uppermost. A chisel that is shaped like a segment of a cylinder with the bevel on the outside is a gouge and can be used to cut a hollow into bone; the bevel prevents the cut from becoming too deep.

An osteotome, designed for making straight cuts through bone is a sharp-edged chisel with bevels on both sides. It is thinner and less robust than a chisel, in order that it does not split the two sides of the cut too widely, and because it does not need to be used with a gouging action. Plan the cut very carefully so that no deviation is necessary.

Chisels and osteotomes are driven through bone using a mallet. This is deliberately short-handled in order to limit the power of each strike. Use this as a reminder that irretrievable damage can be caused to the bone and soft tissues beyond, by ill-considered, badly controlled chisel cuts. Always grasp the chisel firmly with the left hand (Fig. 148) in such a way that the too rapid progression of the cut is prevented. Steady the left hand against the tissues, or brace it by pressing your left elbow into the side of your body.

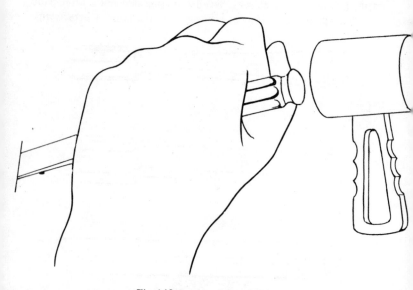

Fig. 148 Cutting with a chisel.

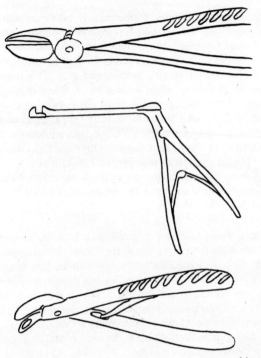

Fig. 149 Bone cutting forceps at top. Rongeurs at centre and bottom.

CUTTING FORCEPS (Fig. 149), acting like scissors, may be used to make small cuts through bone that is not too thick. Remember that these forceps inevitably have a crushing action.

RONGEURS (Fig. 149). Bone may be gnawed or nibbled away with a variety of forceps; inevitably the surface that remains is rather irregular.

Filing

This manoeuvre is much less successful for shaping bone than it is when handling wood and metal. It is limited, as a rule, to rasping the sharp edges from angular cuts made with saws and chisels.

Drilling

This may be carried out using manually operated (Fig. 150) or powered drills. Because the density of bone varies, the rate at which

139

the bit penetrates also varies. Consequently take care when drilling through dense bone, not to lean too heavily upon the drill in case it suddenly breaks through into cancellous bone or soft tissues.

When a carpenter or engineer starts to drill he often indents the surface to start the bit cutting in the right spot. This is usually not convenient to carry out when drilling bone. When drilling into the hard cortex of a round-sectioned long bone, take care in case the drill point 'walks' away from the intended hole, or even slips right off the bone. During the progress of the drill, constantly check that its exit is free from tissues that might be injured. Keep the projecting portion of the bit as short as possible, and protect nearby soft tissues and swabs from getting caught up with the twist bit. Avoid angling the drill, which puts strain upon the bit and may break it.

Screwing

Do not attempt to insert a screw into bone as though it were wood, which usually accepts the extra volume by compacting itself. Cortical bone is too rigid to be compressed in this manner and is likely to split unless a preliminary hole is drilled, which should be the same size as the shank of the screw from which the thread flanges project. Screws used in surgery do not need a thread to be cut for them since they have a self-tapping action.

When fixing long bones, have the screw pierce both cortices, which are dense and give the best grip (Fig. 151). After drilling a hole, estimate its length using a probe or bone depth gauge, and select a screw with a shank this length. The screw may be held initially in a screwdriver that grips its head, but this must be released finally, and the screw is driven home using a conventional screwdriver. Do not overtighten screws, or the grip of the thread is lost.

When using screws to fix plates or other metal fittings, ensure that the metals are compatible. Stainless steel, vitallium and

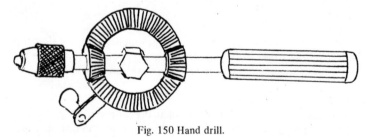

Fig. 150 Hand drill.

tantalum are used. If screws of one metal hold plates of another metal, they generate electrolytic action which weakens the metals and provokes absorption of the bone.

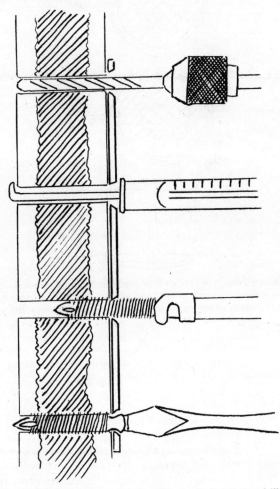

Fig. 151 Plating and screwing long bone. The top hole is being drilled with a twist drill. The next lower hole is being measured with a bone depth gauge. A screw is being inserted into the third hole, held in an automatic screwdriver that grips the screw head. The bottom hole has a fully inserted screw penetrating both cortices.

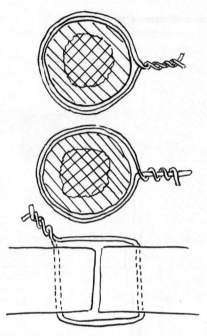

Fig. 152 Wiring bone. Top, the ends of the encircling wire are evenly twisted. Centre, the ends are unevenly twisted and will break, or fail to secure the wire. Bottom, the bone has been drilled so wire can be passed through, like a stitch.

Stitching

Stitches can be inserted into the periosteum or ligaments. Alternatively the bone can be drilled and stitches can then be passed through the holes.

Wiring

Bone may be fixed by encircling it with wire (Fig. 152), the ends of which are then twisted together. Make sure that the wire is not overtightened and weakened at the start of the twist, where it may subsequently break. Ensure that the twisting action is applied equally to the two ends; if one is kept still and the other twisted around it, the twist will not hold, and the spiralled wire will be weakened.

As an alternative to a wire ligature, the bone may be drilled and wire can be passed through the holes

Chapter 8

HANDLING DISPLAY

Surgical procedures can be safely and confidently undertaken only when the tissues are advantageously displayed. Many operations must be carried out in the depths of the wound, where it is difficult to see and manipulate the tissues. There is no merit in overcoming difficulties that can be avoided. Make full use of the available facilities and assistants. Direct others to display and control tissues and instruments that you cannot more ably do yourself, while preventing the help from becoming burdensome.

Incision

Make your incision in the best place to carry out the operation, remembering that the safe, effective accomplishment of the procedure is the prime consideration. Make the incision generous, to provide good access. It is not only the skin incision that must be long enough, but division of the other tissues must match it.

Light

This must be good, even, and free from glare. An overhead source of diffuse light is generally available, so that your head does not produce a shadow. Make sure the lamp is adjusted and focussed correctly. Shiny metal retractors may be used to reflect light into the depths of the wound. Light bulbs on malleable stems, or perspex retractors which direct externally produced light into the depths are sometimes invaluable. When light must be directed down a narrow channel wear a headlamp or a head mirror reflecting light down the hole.

Exteriorize

Bring to the surface of the wound any structure that can be brought there to carry out a delicate procedure. The light, the ability to manipulate, and the freedom from blood collection are better.

143

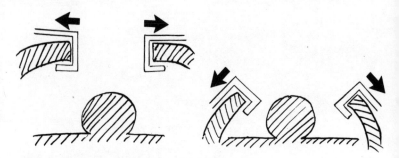

Fig. 153 Displaying a fixed deep structure. Instead of retracting the wound edges, as on the left it may be preferable to depress them as on the right.

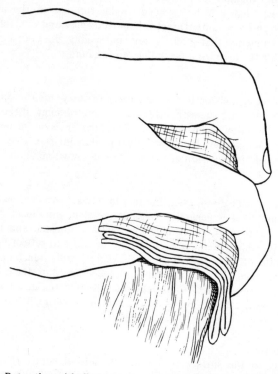

Fig. 154 Retracting with fingers over a gauze swab. The swab gives a better grip of slippery tissues.

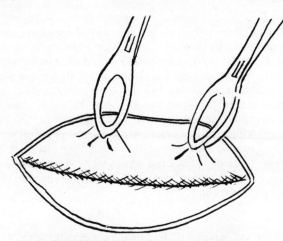

Fig. 155 Using tissue forceps as retractors.

Sometimes the tissue cannot be raised but the wound edges can be depressed (Fig. 153). Sometimes the structure can be raised by placing a pack of gauze behind it.

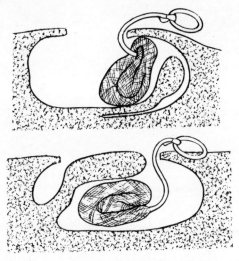

Fig. 156 Using large gauze packs in deep wounds. Top the pack is holding aside a structure. Bottom the pack is lifting a structure into the wound.

Retraction

The wound edges and overlying or attached structures must be carefully displaced to provide a good view. Self-retaining wound retractors (Fig. 13) may free the assistant to help in other ways but they overstretch and damage the wound edges if they are roughly opened. Hand-held retractors can be constantly adjusted by an intelligent assistant, who relaxes the pull between procedures. Overlying structures can be displaced with fingers (Fig. 154), swabs, tissue forceps (Fig. 155) or traction sutures. Large packs, suitably attached by tapes so that they cannot be inadvertently left in the wound, may be used to hold out of the way loose structures that tend to obscure the field of operation and to lift other structures into the wound (Fig. 156).

Haemostasis

Prevention and control of bleeding are essential for careful and deliberate surgery. If the field is obscured by blood the surgical assessment will be sketchy, and the operation will be haphazard.

Chapter 9

HANDLING DISSECTION

Objects
 Dissection of tissue may be necessary to approach a structure in order to identify it, examine it, or display it. A structure may require dissecting free in order to carry out a procedure upon it, or to excise it. Surgical dissection is carried out with the minimum trauma and disturbance of structures.

Sharp dissection
SCALPEL. The scalpel divides tissues with minimal damage. Select this method when the anatomical features are confidently known, and when the tissues are homogeneous. The scalpel divides tissues cleanly only when they can resist the frictional drag of the knife blade. Sometimes they must be held under tension to produce sufficient resistance. If tension can be applied at right angles to the direction of the incision, the tissues separate and reveal the deeper structures (Fig. 157).
SCISSORS. Expertly performed scissors dissection produces minimal

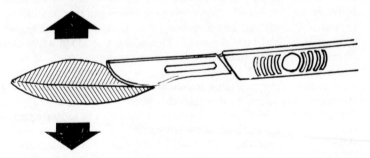

Fig. 157 If tension is applied at right angles to the incision while cutting, the depths of the incision are immediately visible.

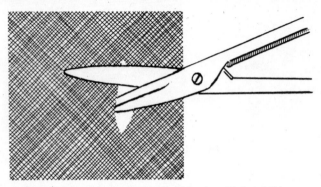

Fig. 158 When cutting with scissors the deep blade is hidden.

tissue damage. The blades must remain rigidly in contact with each other while cutting, or the tissues will be crushed, not cut. A potential danger with scissors dissection is that the deep blade is hidden from view while it is cutting (Fig. 158). Anticipate this and identify the whole thickness of the tissue before cutting it. An advantage offered by scissors is that they may be used both for sharp and blunt dissection.

DIATHERMY. A steady oscillating diathermy current applied through a pointed active electrode, disrupts the tissues. At the same time the cut surface is partially coagulated so that small blood vessels are sealed. Cutting diathermy is particularly useful when dividing large masses of vascular soft tissue, such as muscle.

Blunt dissection
SPLITTING. Muscles, some aponeuroses, the connective tissue close to linear structures such as blood vessels, nerves and tendons, can be separated by splitting. The direction of the fibres follows the line of greatest tension within the body. This is the line along which the fibres may be split, since there are fewer connecting fibres at right angles to the line of tension. Scissors can be used to split a sheet after it has been penetrated in one place, and separated from deep structures. Insert one blade of an almost closed scissors through the hole. Push the scissors in the direction of the fibres to separate them. (Fig. 159). When there are some strong fibres at right angles to the main line of fibres, the sharp edges of the blades cut through them.

An entirely different splitting action may be achieved with scissors. Hold them perpendicular to the plane of the tissues. Push

148

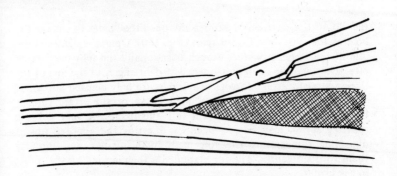

Fig. 159 Splitting parallel fibres with scissors. The scissors are almost closed. The small 'V' between the blade tips is pushed in the line of the fibres.

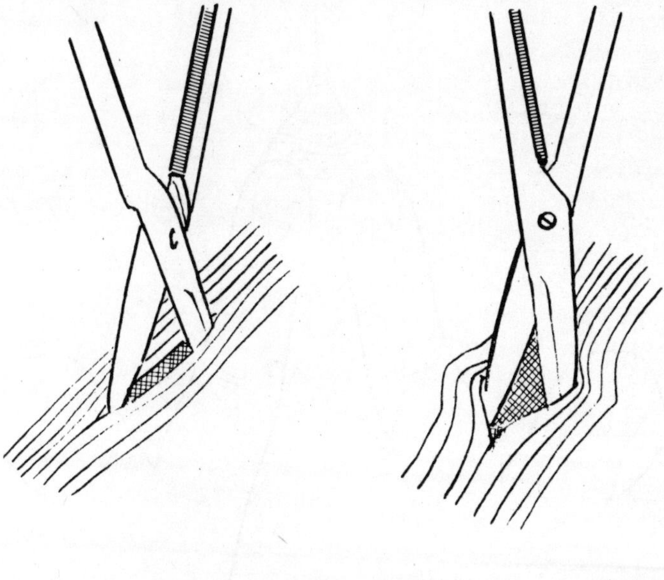

Fig. 160 Splitting parallel fibres with scissors. The closed tips are pushed into the sheet of fibres and then opened. On the left the blades are opened parallel to the fibres, on the right they are opened at right angles to the fibres.

the closed tips between the fibres and open the blades to enlarge the hole as the fibres are forced apart (Fig. 160). Open the blades in the line of the fibres as a rule, though occasionally the splitting is more effective when the blades are opened at right angles to the line of the fibres. Straight artery forceps of suitable size may be used instead of scissors (Figs. 92, 93). The rounded backs of the artery forceps blades have less tendency to cut into the tissues. A very delicate splitting action may be produced by inserting the apposed tips of dissecting forceps into the hole made in the tissues, and allowing them to open gently. The force applied is then limited by the spring in the blades.

The splitting action may be accomplished by inserting two fingers into a hole in the tissue sheet, and then separating the fingers. Splitting may be carried out using one finger, the handle of a scalpel or similar instrument, and sweeping it along in the line of the desired split. For the stripping of periosteum from bone, special instruments are available. They are pushed or pulled in contact with the bone and cleanly split off the periosteum.

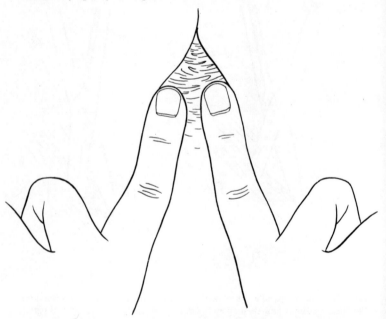

Fig. 161 Tearing tissues to separate them, opening up a plane of cleavage.

TEARING. This method sounds crude and traumatic and so it can be when used inappropriately or roughly. Selection depends on your judgment of the relative strengths of the tissues. If two pieces of joined tissue are pulled apart with fingers or forceps, a tear will occur in the weakest tissue (Fig. 161). When using this method, keep careful watch to ensure that the line of the tear does not deviate from the selected path. The presence of disease may weaken structures considered to be strong.

WIPING. A finger, bluntnosed dissecting forceps, a knife handle, or a gauze swab can be used to wipe one tissue from another and separate them (Fig. 162). The force is limited by frictional contact between the wiping instrument and the tissues. Powerful traction may be exerted with a dry gauze swab. Wiping is appropriately used to separate two structures diffusely joined by flimsy connective tissue,

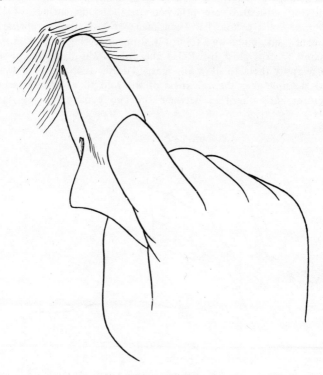

Fig. 162 Wiping. A finger wrapped in a gauze swab wipes the tissues apart.

and to detach areolar tissue from a structure in order to display it. Filmy connective fibres are broken down with most gentle wiping action but stronger fibres may need additional judicious sharp dissection. Remember that rubbing the tissues is very damaging to them. Wiping does not imply attempts to wear through connective tissue.

PINCHING. Circumscribed attachment of two structures may be broken down if it is compressed, provided the attachment is weaker than the structures it joins together. Compression may be achieved by squeezing the attachment between finger and thumb (Fig. 163).

Selection of methods

MEMBRANOUS TISSUES. When penetrating a membranous layer avoid damaging underlying structures. It is impossible to be sure if underlying structures are attached to the deep surface of the membrane until a hole has been made in it. If the membrane is sufficiently lax, pinch up a fold of it, using dissecting forceps. Apply a second forceps close by. Relax the grip of the first forceps and then re-apply them to allow any grasped deep structure to fall away. When possible feel the thickness of the fold to exclude attached structures. Lift the fold between the two pairs of forceps, and

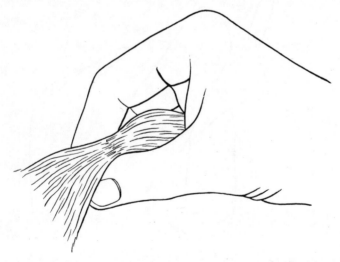

Fig. 163 Pinching a segment of tissue between finger and thumb to break it down through its weakest part.

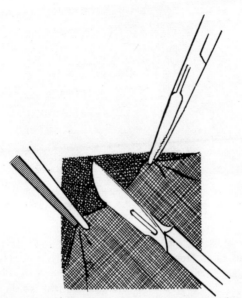

Fig. 164 Making an initial incision through a membrane, after lifting a ridge with forceps.

carefully incise the ridge of membrane with a scalpel (Fig. 164). Remove the forceps and explore the deep surface of the membrane through the hole. If the membrane is taut, or adherent to deeper structures, it cannot be tented. Incise the layer using light strokes with the belly of the scalpel blade. If possible, apply tension on each side at right angles to the line of incision, to separate the edges so that the depth of remaining tissue can be estimated.

Through the entry hole assess the presence of deep attachments. Insert the blades of dissecting forceps or two fingers to feel through the hole. Use the forceps (Fig. 165) or two fingers to separate the deep surface of the membrane from other structures and cut between the forceps blades or fingers using a scalpel or scissors, depending on the direction of the cut. As the incision is enlarged it becomes progressively easier to inspect the deep aspect of the membrane.

When it is critically important not to penetrate deeper than the chosen layer, try infiltrating it with isotonic saline solution to expand the tissues and render them translucent. As structures are approached, they can be seen before they are cut.

153

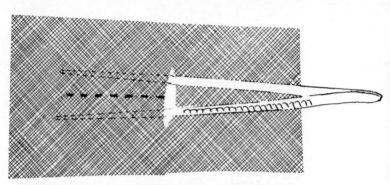

Fig. 165 To enlarge a hole through a membranous layer, insert dissecting forceps through the hole and incise the membrane between the blades of the forceps as indicated by the dotted line.

SHEETS OF VASCULAR CONNECTIVE TISSUE. If the sheet contains a few large blood vessels, display, isolate, doubly clamp, divide and ligate them before attempting to divide the rest of the membrane (Fig. 166). If the sheet contains many smaller vessels,

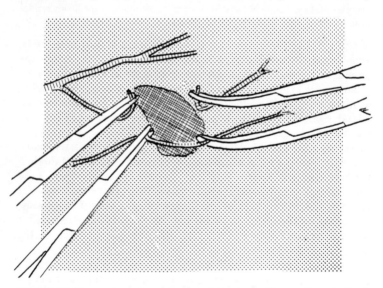

Fig. 166 Dividing a sheet of vascular connective tissue. The vessels are isolated and divided between clamps before incising the sheet of tissue.

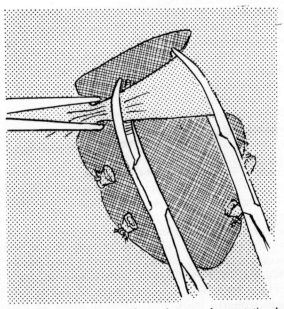

Fig. 167 Dividing vascular membrane between haemostatic clamps. The forceps on the right will not grip the full width of flattened ribbon of membrane. On the left the portion of membrane has been bunched with dissecting forceps before clamping it. Note that the left hand forceps will have tips projecting beyond the clamped membrane, to facilitate ligation.

apply artery forceps in pairs, one on each side of the proposed line of section, and cut between them. Do not attempt to gather too much tissue into the forceps, or they will slip. Artery forceps grasp only near their tips. Do not expect them to grip a wide flat sheet; bunch the tissue first (Fig. 167). Make sure the tips of the forceps project beyond the tissue, so that it can be ligated easily. If the tissue contains only a few minor blood vessels, divide it with scalpel or scissors, picking up the blood vessels individually for ligation or diathermy coagulation. When possible, pick up vessels before cutting them.

When dividing a very vascular membrane, try infiltrating it first with isotonic saline containing adrenaline in a concentration of 1/400,000; this causes vasoconstriction and reduces oozing. Alternatively use diathermy cutting current judiciously.

HOMOGENEOUS TISSUES. Clean cuts with the belly of a sharp

155

scalpel divide soft tissues with minimal damage. If possible, apply tension on each side at right angles to the line of the incision to open it up. The tissues separate as they are divided, making it easier to assess the depth of the cut. Scratch-like cuts make the edges of the wound ragged and small pieces of tissue are deprived of blood supply. Make each successive cut along the line of the preceding one, in the deepest part of the wound.

The fibres in homogenous tissue are sometimes aligned in one direction. In muscles, and frequently in connective tissues, instead of cutting across the fibres, whenever possible try to split between them.

If an important linear structure such as a nerve, blood vessel, tendon, or duct may be encountered, cut parallel to its expected course. As a safeguard, the tissues may be artificially split into successive layers thin enough to identify structures within them. As each successive layer is demonstrated to be free of important structures, divide it. Create the layers by inserting the blades of closed scissors, artery forceps, or non-toothed dissecting forceps, angling the blades to lie parallel to the surface, and then gently open them to form a track. Confirm that the layer is safe to cut. When using scissors withdraw them, insert one blade along the track, and divide the layer. When using forceps leave them in place, and cut between the opened blades with scalpel or scissors. Proceed now to separate another layer, and continue in this way until the sought-after structure is reached.

When penetrating homogeneous tissue in search of a structure, the safest technique may be a combination of splitting and tearing. Hold scissors, artery forceps, or dissecting forceps with closed blades, perpendicular to the surface. Push in the points to create a hole, and open the blades to tear the tissues apart. If scissors are used a rapid, effective, but potentially dangerous combination of blunt and sharp dissection is possible. Remember also that very powerful pressure is exerted at the tips of artery forceps or scissors blades when they are forcibly opened, and tissues may be indiscriminately disrupted.

DISEASED TISSUES. The fibrous tissue laid down in response to many disease processes is often irregular and opaque so there may be no warning of impending trouble. The connective tissue sheath that normally encloses many important structures may be destroyed by disease. The structure may be suddenly exposed and inadvertently damaged. Disease often alters the character of the tissues so that a structure is not recognized. Also, the anatomical features may be destroyed or distorted by the disease process.

Remember that the differential strengths of tissues may be changed by disease processes. Tearing, splitting, wiping or pinching depend upon the fact that some structures are stronger and more resistant to the forces employed than others. Before exerting any force in the presence of disease, make sure the force will not disrupt a vital structure. Structures which are easily swept aside in normal conditions may be adherent, thickened, and resistant to blunt dissection, so that sharp dissection must be resorted to, with the attendant risks.

Whenever possible start a dissection away from the diseased area, recognize the tissues where they are relatively normal and then work towards the diseased area, maintaining exposure of important structures throughout.

Some neoplasms and chronically inflamed tissues must be excised through normal tissues, avoiding contact with the surface of the structure. This demands the greatest degree of skill and caution. In addition to the demands of a technique which precludes confirmation of the anatomy by reference to the surface of the part to be excised, the surrounding tissues may be distorted and changed in character by the disease. Learn to recognize diseased tissue, know its likely confines, and the local anatomy. Decide what structures must be spared and what may be sacrificed.

Aids

ANATOMY. Learn the anatomy of the part because it is vital to performing safe and effective dissection. This knowledge must include not only the situation of the structures but also their appearance, texture, and relative strengths; it must include not only the normal anatomy but also a knowledge of the variations which may occur.

PALPATION. If an important structure is likely to be palpable, feel for it before starting, and at each step in the dissection. Feel for arterial pulsations but remember that tension obliterates them. Feel in the expected situation, and in the surroundings if the structure could be misplaced. If it is hard, it may be sought with the point of a sharp needle. If it is a duct or vessel containing fluid, search for it with a hollow needle and attached syringe, so the fluid can be aspirated to identify it.

FLUID INFILTRATION. If the tissues are infiltrated with isotonic

157

saline they swell and this facilitates the separation of structures. The fluid renders the tissues more transparent so that structures are seen before they are reached. The turgidity braces the tissues against the frictional drag of cutting instruments. Fluid spreads easily in the tissue planes, facilitating dissection along these paths. The pressure of fluid reduces bleeding, but adrenaline, 1 part in 400,000 may be added, to produce vasoconstriction.

TRANSILLUMINATION. Sometimes the structures can be lifted and viewed against the light, or a light can be placed behind them.

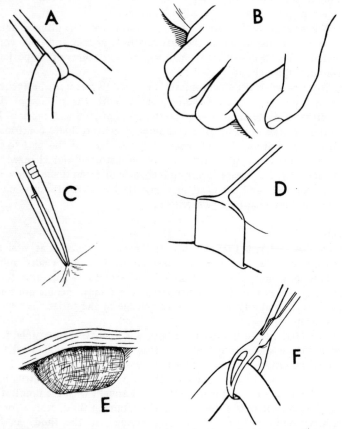

Fig. 168 Methods of exerting traction. A, Tape. B, Hand. C, Dissecting forceps. D, Retractor. E, Packs. F, Tissue forceps.

Structures can thus be identified—but remember that compressed and emptied veins may transilluminate and so be inadvertently damaged. Always try to relax the tissues when transilluminating them.

TENSION. Correctly applied tension aids successful dissection. Straighten and slightly stretch relaxed or folded tissues that are to be incised. Stretching thins the tissue, allowing approached structures to be identified early, since most normal tissues in the body are partially translucent. If possible, view the stretched tissues against the light, but remember to relax the tension to allow emptied veins to fill and so become visible.

When tissues are to be cut, tension helps to fix them so that they do not slip away from the cutting force. Moreover, the incision passes through the minimum amount of tissue. As the incision is made, tension may be applied to retract the cut surfaces, exposing the deeper, uncut parts.

Apply tension by pulling or lifting one structure away from another. Exert traction with the hands, tissue forceps, dissecting forceps, swabs, tapes, or retractors (Fig. 168). Maintain it by using self-retaining retractors, packs, and when appropriate, gravity.

Do not rely upon steady, unremitting traction. Tension distorts the relationships between structures. It obliterates palpable arterial pulsations that warn of the presence of the vessels. Frequently relax the tissues to allow them to return to their normal position and re-assess them to prevent errors. Apply tension in different directions from time to time to ensure that the best direction is selected.

STAY IN THE CORRECT PLANE. Once the surface of an important structure has been identified in the correct plane, do not leave it. If the dissection is allowed to wander away from its surface, the structure is endangered because it cannot be seen. Can the structure be moved from its surroundings, or can the surroundings be moved, to tense and display the junctional tissues, allowing accurate dissection in the correct plane?

The tissues adjoining the surface of the structure to be displayed may be split in a direction parallel to the surface or at right angles to it. A firm tough structure, such as a bone, is able to withstand the pressure of one blade of the forceps, so that they may be opened at right angles to it. Near a structure that may have branches, such as a blood vessel, also split at right angles to the surface; any damage is immediately visible. Splitting in the line of the vessel may tear off the origins of branches.

BE FLEXIBLE. Do not inexorably display structures from one aspect. Make a fresh approach from another direction if the dissection becomes difficult. If the application of tension, or the retraction of other structures alters the anatomical situation, restore the structures to their original situation at frequent intervals to confirm the relationships between them.

Do not be limited in your technique. A combination of blunt and sharp dissection is often required. Use blunt dissection, whether it be by splitting, wiping, tearing or pinching, until the areas requiring sharp dissection have been defined. Then, after re-assessment, resort to knife or scissors.

KEEP THE FIELD FREE OF BLOOD. Bleeding is inimical to safe effective dissection. Prevent potential bleeding, control it when it occurs, and remove blood that collects as a result of bleeding. Working in the depths, in the midst of pooled blood with continuing, uncontrolled bleeding, is a certain recipe for disaster.

Dissecting round structures

It is frequently necessary to dissect behind a large structure, either to secure the blood vessels entering the structure before excising it, or to carry out a procedure on another structure hidden behind the mass.

Do not perform this difficult manoeuvre unless it is really necessary. Sometimes a change in the direction of approach will allow you to reach the area of dissection directly. Sometimes the mass can be diminished in size; for instance a large cyst can be aspirated of fluid and thus collapsed.

Whenever you cannot avoid dissecting behind a large structure, keep as flexible an attitude as possible throughout the dissection. Do not proceed doggedly if the going becomes hazardous, or you may make an error. Immediately stop and approach from another direction. Make sure that you have sufficient light, draw the structure aside when possible, and make sure that it is mobilized fully. Ensure that the approach is the best possible, that the incision is generous, and that other structures that obscure the view have been moved aside.

Remember that such a dissection is at its most difficult at the start, and becomes progressively easier. The moments of danger are at the beginning, when a mistake prejudices the whole of the rest of the dissection, and at the end when overconfidence may spoil a previously painstaking dissection.

160

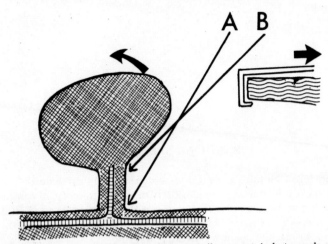

Fig. 169 The base of the pedicle is most easily seen at A, but vessels can be better controlled if they are first sought at B.

Choose to start the dissection where you get the best view, where you are most clear about the anatomical relationships, where you can best control major blood vessels and where a minor division of tissue is most likely to facilitate further dissection. Of course all these aims are unlikely to be met at any one point, so start at the point that offers the best compromise but review the approach during the rest of the dissection.

If you are deprived of a view, make as much use as possible of your sense of feel, palpating structures and testing their strength. Remember when feeling for arterial pulsations that tension will obliterate the pulsation, so relax the structure while palpating it.

Do not cut blindly. This rule almost never requires to be broken. Do not cut until you have taken every precaution to control unexpected bleeding; this may be achieved by grasping a vascular pedicle between finger and thumb, placing a clamp, ready to close, across the pedicle, or encircling it with a tape or ligature, ready to be tightened. When transecting a pedicle, remember that although it may be initially easier to cut as far away from the structure as possible, this will make the remaining pedicle shorter and more difficult to control (Fig. 169).

Finally, remember to worry about problems in the correct order. The first problem is not 'How shall I carry out this dissection?' but 'How shall I best approach this dissection?'

Chapter 10

HANDLING BLEEDING

Uncontrolled bleeding is dangerous because it may cause death, but apart from this dramatic conclusion it may lead to hasty, ill-considered actions that prejudice the success of the surgical procedure. If it continues after the operation is completed it may still kill the patient, or mar the operative result.

Prevention

Make sure that the subject has no correctable bleeding tendency or anaemia beforehand. Learn the anatomy, remembering that congenital anomalies and disease processes may confound your expectations. Whenever possible display major blood vessels and obtain control by getting an assistant to hold them between finger and thumb ready to compress them, or apply an open, non-crushing clamp across them, ready to be closed (Fig. 112), or encircle them with thread or tape, the end of the tape being led through a length of rubber tubing to form a snare which can be tightened and clamped if necessary (Fig. 114).

If major blood vessels have to be divided, display and control them first, to guard against premature injury to them. Apply clamps on each side of the point of division, section the vessels (Fig. 70), and then ligate them. Alternatively pass two ligatures using an aneurysm needle (Fig. 72), tie them well clear of the point of section and then divide the vessels. Very large vessels should be doubly ligated, or closed with suture-ligatures (Fig. 74).

If vascular tissues must be divided, try to control the supplying vessels. If this is not possible have an assistant compress the tissues, or apply a non-crushing clamp on either side of the line of section. Sometimes a constricting stitch may be placed and tied on each side, parallel to the cut. (Fig. 143).

When preliminary control cannot be achieved before sectioning

162

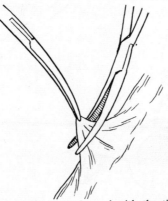

Fig. 170 A bleeding vessel has been clamped with the tip of the left hand forceps. The forceps are gently pulled upon to tent the area while a second forceps is applied with points projecting, to facilitate ligating it.

vascular tissues, try dividing them with the diathermy current applied through a needle, using a steady oscillating current, which has a localized cutting effect, switching to a damped current to coagulate individual bleeding vessels. Sometimes vascular tissues can be separated bluntly, so that large buried vessels can be identified and controlled. Do not allow bleeding to get out of hand, but stop and control it. Occasionally a bold division may facilitate efficient haemostasis.

Be doubly careful when working in the depths. It is difficult to obtain a good view, and any oozed blood collects over the bleeding vessel and obscures it.

Take care when dissecting near venous sinuses that may be held open by surrounding structures. Beware of large veins near the heart that may channel air into the heart and cause frothing, with immediate circulatory failure.

In certain circumstances preliminary infiltration of the area with physiological saline containing 1 part of adrenaline in 400,000 prevents oozing by constricting the blood vessels. Cooling the tissues also reduces vascularity.

Control

Once bleeding occurs from isolated vessels, pick them up with haemostatic forceps for subsequent ligature, or diathermization. The initial haemostatic forceps may offer no tip projecting beyond the

163

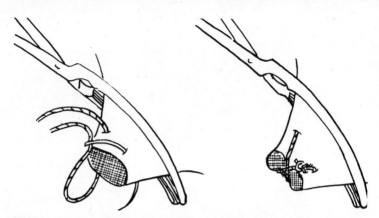

Fig. 171 If a cut vessel retracts into the tissue, compress but do not crush the tissues. A non-crushing clamp has been applied in the diagrams. On the left a double stitch has been inserted and tied on the right to control bleeding.

vessel to hold down the loop of a ligature; do not hesitate to apply a second forceps deep to it, with tip projecting (Fig. 170). Generalized oozing can be staunched by pressure from a gauze pack, compressing the area manually, with a retractor, or by trapping the pack under the wound edge.

If a major vessel is inadvertently divided, control it initially by direct pressure, or by compressing a main feeding vessel. Do not act rashly. It may be possible, or even essential to repair the vessel. Do not compound the error by damaging other structures. Remember that bleeding is usually worst at the moment it starts and time is on your side. If you feel shaken, maintain control and do no more until your equanimity has returned; by this time the bleeding will have stopped or diminished. Trying to grab a major blood vessel in a pool of blood will end in disaster. If bleeding can be controlled for five minutes, the problem becomes less frightening.

ARTERIAL bleeding may be dramatic but is usually not worrrying. Nearly all cut arteries will contract after a few minutes, often enough to stop the bleeding altogether. Few arteries are absolutely essential to normal life, and those that are can usually be repaired.

If the artery is buried in other tissues, and retracts, it may be controlled by compressing the whole tissue using a non-crushing clamp, fingers or pressure against a firm structure. The vessel can then be dissected out, clamped and ligated. Alternatively, a stitch may be passed through the tissue twice and then ligated, the double thread constricting the tissues containing the cut vessel (Fig. 171).

VENOUS bleeding may be difficult to control. Oozing from retracted veins between serous membranes may form an enlarging haematoma with separation of the layers. Clamping and ligation, or suture ligation reduces the oozing from the edge while the uncontrolled vessel continues to bleed, increasing the size of the haematoma. Do not waste time trying to pick up the vessel. Place a curved non-crushing clamp or swab-holding forceps over the proximal part of the haematoma, and leave it in place for as long as possible.

Deep venous oozing bleeds frighteningly, the dark blood welling up into the wound. Do not attempt to clamp the invisible vessel but pack the depths for at least 5 minutes, timed by the clock. Make sure you have controlled the bleeding before waiting. When you remove the pack, the bleeding may well have stopped. Do not hesitate in hazardous situations to leave part of a long roll of gauze packing the area, taking the end out through the wound, to be removed in a couple of days.

Beware of venous sinuses running in rigid structures, that prevent them from collapsing when they are cut. If you can control the bleeding with local pressure it may be possible to repair the vein, or to place stitches round it to ligate it. Take extra care when operating in the region of major central veins. If they are inadvertently opened, they may suck in air that foams in the blood within the heart, and instantly halts the circulation.

CAPILLARY oozing is not usually a problem. It can be controlled by gentle pressure, or applying heat in the form of diathermy or hot wet gauze packs. If capillary oozing continues from an extensive area, pick up each small bleeding vessel to twist it, ligate it or diathermize it. Always work from above downwards, to avoid obscuring the field with blood dripping over the area. Sometimes the whole area can be successfully compressed with packs, non-crushing clamps, or stitches. The raw area of a viscus may be folded and stitched upon itself to compress oozing vessels. Gelatine foam or a portion of excised and crushed muscle may be sewn over the area to promote clotting.

Appendix

ANATOMICAL TERMS

Since the use of these terms is economical and adds to the accuracy of the descriptions, they are defined for those who are unfamiliar with them.

The body is considered to be erect, arms hanging, palms facing forward. The midline between the left and right halves is the *median plane*. A plane parallel to this is referred to as the *sagittal plane*. A vertical plane at right angles to the median plane is the *coronal plane*. A plane at right angles to the median and coronal planes is a *horizontal plane*.

The front of the body is called *anterior* or *ventral*, the back of the body is *posterior* or *dorsal*. The upper part of the body is *superior* or *cephalic* and lower part *inferior*, or *caudal*.

Especially in the limbs, *proximal* is used to describe a part near the body, *distal* is used to describe a part away from the body. In the hand, *palmar* is used as an alternative to anterior. In the foot, *plantar* is used as an alternative for the sole of the foot.

Medial describes a structure near the midline of the body, *lateral* describes a structure away from the midline. When describing the hand, the lateral edge also called the radial edge, is the thumb edge, the medial edge also called the ulnar edge, is the little finger edge. For individual fingers, the same terms are used. The medial edge of the middle finger normally lies in contact with the ring finger, the lateral edge contacts the index fingers.

External denotes near the surface, *internal* is reserved for the inside of body cavities. *Superficial* means near the body surface, *deep* means far from the body surface.

The individual segments of the fingers are the *phalanges*, (singular *phalanx*) and the joints are the *interphalangeal* joints. The knuckle joints are the *metacarpophalangeal* joints.

The soft, fleshy, palmar surface covering each terminal phalanx will be referred to as the *pulp* of the finger.

Flexion is the bending of a joint to approximate the parts which it connects. The fingers are flexed when making a fist. The opposite movement is that of *extension*.

Apposition of surfaces has a special meaning in the hand when the thumb pulp is apposed to the pulps of the fingers, since the thumb rotates in its long axis.

Pronation is the movement of face or palm downwards. The reverse movement, turning the palm or face upwards, is *supination*.

Abduction is movement of a limb from the median plane of the body, *adduction* is movement towards the median plane. In the hand, finger movements are referred to the median plane of the arm continued along the centre of the middle finger. Movement of other digits away from the middle finger is abduction, movement towards the middle finger is adduction. Lateral movement of the middle finger in either direction is abduction.

INDEX